How the Doctors Diet

How the Doctors Diet

PETER AND BARBARA WYDEN

Trident Press, New York

Preface

Doctors are notoriously busy people. They are also traditionally reluctant to talk about themselves. In this book 89 doctors and their families nevertheless disclose more (and more intimate) information about themselves than has ever been made public before. We are convinced that they took time out to do this for only one reason: their genuine concern for your health. It's a refreshing thing to think about, and we would like to thank them on behalf of our readers.

Peter and Barbara Wyden

CONTENTS

1 *Yes, There is a Doctors' Diet* 11

2 DR. MAYER : *The Gourmet Who Wants To Live Forever* 17

3 DR. STARE : *Swallowing His Own Medicine* 29

4 THE ALEXANDERS : *Two Experts in the Family* 42

5 DR. STAMLER : *Gluttony Under Control* 49

6 DR. WHITE : *Staying Trim Under Pressure* 58

7 DR. BRUCE TAYLOR : *An Extremist for Good Reason* 67

8 DR. RUBIN : *The Formerly Fat Psychiatrist* 74

9 DR. COHN : *Life Is Just a Bowl of Nibbles* 84

10 DR. PAGE : *An Elder Statesman's Diet* 92

11 DR. ANCEL KEYS : *Eating Lean, the High-Style Way* 104

12 DR. FRANTZ : *A Physician in Search of a Cure* 114

13 DR. BROWN : *When You Really Love Good Food* 121

14 DR. HELLERSTEIN : *Impatient Apostle of Exercise* 126

15 DR. BERMAN : *The Reluctant Revolutionary* 138

16 DR. HARRIS : *Feeling Guilty* 144

17 DR. "SMITH" : *How To Succeed at Dieting Without Really Thinking* 150

18 DR. HUNDLEY : *A Will of Iron—and a Stomach to Match* 157

19 DR. MUNVES : *Living It Up on Weekends* 164

20 DR. CHRISTAKIS : *Chief of the Prudent Dieters* 173

21 DR. RINZLER : *Confessions of a Cake Eater* 184

22 DR. SCHILLING : *Stopping Trouble Before It Starts* 192

23 DR. GLENN : *The Reform School that Gets Results* 201

24 *How Doctors Diet* 209

25 *Living with the Doctors' Diet* 240
    Index 252

1

Yes, There Is a Doctors' Diet

This is a book of ready-to-use facts, not suppositions, but at the outset it seems reasonably safe to venture one guess: The fact that you have picked up this volume suggests that you are one of the 79 million American adults—about half of a nation—who are overweight; or one of the 42,500,000 who are actively concerned about their waistlines; or even one of the 9,500,000 who are actually on a weight-reducing diet right now. And if you are indeed a member of this vast and affluent club, the chances are also excellent that you have wondered how the other half lives—the more or less equally prosperous, yet trim, lean other half of a nation.

We happen to be in a good position to sympathize with you because both of us have been overweight for more years than we care to recall and we have always been envious of everybody who is not. After several years of research into our affliction we have begun to concede, however grudgingly, that the vast majority of these other Americans—the attractively trim ones—are not really very different from our- selves except in one respect: They eat less than we do, and most of them somehow get more exercise.

Clearly, these are very fortunate people. In today's society, thinness has become a much-envied status sym- bol, and these people have attained it; they can there- fore lord it over the rest of us, and they often do. Secondly, we all know that thinness is almost a requirement if you are even the least bit vain and like to fit into the snug, revealing clothes that fashion increasingly prescribes for women and, more recently, even for men. Thirdly, there can no longer be any doubt that thinness is nothing more nor less than a strategic preventive against our No. 1 killer—heart and artery disease.

All right, so the stakes are high. In point of fact, there is little we overweight Americans can do in our own self-interest that is more important than to find out all we can about the trim Americans. How *do* they do it? How do they subdue their hunger pangs? How do they manage to skimp on their favorite foods and drinks? How do they contrive to exert themselves physically when they, like the rest of us, don't really have to? Do these seemingly privileged citizens actually have any secrets? And if they do, can we find out what they are and make use of them ourselves?

This book will answer these questions. Our evidence will come from the most reliable and professional witnesses who can be summoned to testify. These are the experts who—unlike most dieters—know how to report on their eating and exercise habits with the honesty and precision required by their profession: the doctors who spend their lives trying to persuade others to take off weight.

We had met a lot of these men and their families before we began working on this report. As a group, they were about the trimmest people we knew. They were also among the most accommodating. And so we went to them with a request nobody had made before.

"Don't tell us what you want us to do about our weight and exercise," we said. "Tell us *what you do yourselves*, and what your families do, to get trim and stay that way."

We made this request to 89 leading diet specialists, wherever they practice throughout the nation—at the most prestigious universities, hospitals and clinics, at government agencies and professional societies. Every member of the elite American Society for Clinical Nutrition was also questioned. We talked personally not only to many of these doctors but also to their wives and to some of their children. Just about without exception, they were a marvelously cooperative group. Generously they agreed to open up their caloric private lives (and sometimes even their refrigerators) for our inspection. The results surprised us, and they add up to what may well be today's biggest unreported diet news.

What we discovered is something that we had long suspected but that had never been documented: namely, that for many years there has actually existed a regimen that can fairly be called "The Doctors' Diet." It is not a pat formula. In fact, it is a surprisingly casual affair. What is of singular importance to you and to us is that it maximizes the chances for a trim figure, for more vigorous health and for longer life. We think it's high time the rest of us knew all about it.

The doctors arrived at their diet gradually, usually within the past ten years or so. Many of them found it advisable to refine it further in the past few years as the results of new research began to appear in medical journals. As they devised ways to apply this research profitably to themselves, many—probably most—of the best-informed physicians and nutritionists quietly made further substantial changes in the way they eat, drink and live. Often these changes were made quite recently, and here is something else that ought to concern us: With the rarest of exceptions, these doctors were nowhere near as urgently in need of making these changes as the rest of us. Almost all of them now weigh less than they did some years ago, but most of them were pretty lean to begin with, and almost none suffered from such complications as elevated blood pressure or above-normal blood cholesterol levels.

In other words, these doctors started out as better health risks than most of us. Yet they changed their food and exercise patterns because they had become convinced that it was just plain good sense for them and for their families to do so. We will analyze their new patterns here, including the way these experts' wives shop, cook and feed their children.

We found this, frankly, an absolutely fascinating story, and we will use three methods to report it so that not a single useful element will be lost to you, the ordinary dieter:

First, we will visit the homes of twenty-two of

these doctors and their families and will report on their eating and exercise habits in case-by-case, step-by-step clinical detail.

Second, we will draw out of these case histories the highlights of what we learned from our experts and summarize their twelve key diet-and-exercise milestones for you.

Third, we will discuss how you can live with the Doctors' Diet.

We were tempted to call this book "The Thinking Man's Diet" because our doctors remained true to their promise to give us only facts—no lectures. Not one will issue instructions. They will merely let you in on what they think is best for themselves, for their wives and for their children. The rest is entirely up to you.

2

DR. MAYER : *The Gourmet Who Wants To Live Forever*

No diet history fascinated us more than that of Dr. Jean Mayer. He is, first of all, one of the most distinguished researchers and educators in the entire specialty of investigating the causes and cures of overweight. He has written more than three hundred scientific papers on diet and exercise. Some of medicine's most revealing recent findings on such basic human functions as appetite, satiety and body composition have come out of his laboratory at the Harvard University School of Public Health, where Dr.

Mayer is a physiologist and professor of nutrition. He is one of the most influential and widely quoted experts in his field. The phrase, "rhythm method of girth control," often used to describe the up-and-down cycle of many dieters' feast-and-famine habits, was coined by him.

But Dr. Mayer is also refreshingly different as a person. He is what the French call a *type*. In fact, he has all the charm, irreverence and loquacity of a born Frenchman, which he is, and his reputation for caustic candor is deserved. Moreover, we had already known him long enough to realize that Dr. Mayer is a gourmet with a weight problem. So we anticipated the doctor's dietary confessions with particular curiosity. He didn't let us down.

A restless, small, but broad-shouldered man, Dr. Mayer measures five feet seven inches and checks his weight once a week. When we talked with him, he was forty-six and weighed 147 pounds.

"That's more than I think I should," he told us, speaking rapidly and with a strong French accent. "I want to weigh about a hundred forty-two. Anything between a hundred forty and a hundred fifty pounds is perfectly satisfactory, but I'd rather be in the lower range. A couple of years ago I was down to a hundred forty and a half. I've been as high as a hundred sixty-five in very bad winters when I got no exercise at all. I was ashamed of myself."

In the past few years Dr. Mayer has coped successfully with his gourmet tastes, and while he doesn't count calories literally, he estimates he eats no more than two thousand or so a day. He conceded that a certain amount of constant self-discipline is necessary to keep his weight down and that it's never easy.

"There are never days when I eat as much as I could," he said. "I just decide when I've had enough. Rousseau said hygiene is a virtue more than a science. I don't think you can be healthy without some self-denial." Unquestionably, the doctor's willpower is continually recharged by his daily contact with new diet research, especially the increasingly persuasive statistical documentation that overweight and excessive intake of fat, especially animal fat, tend to shorten life. Dr. Mayer, who has worked with laboratory animals as well as thousands of human subjects in New England and in Europe, has himself contributed an impressive portion of this new evidence.

"I have no doubt that overweight is bad," he said. "Ten percent is bad; twenty percent is very bad; thirty percent is extremely bad."

Whatever weight problem Dr. Mayer does have, he attributes to his sedentary life. "It's entirely the result of the nature of my job," he said. "It's intellectually satisfying, but it's not what I ought to be doing physically."

This is an almost unanimous complaint among our doctors, just as it is for almost all time-conscious American business and professional men, and Dr. Mayer happens to be even busier than most. He runs his laboratory with the grace and application of a benevolent despot. He teaches not only nutrition but is proud to be the only professor at Harvard to give a course in the history of medicine. He is always in the middle of a scientific paper and for years has been working on a book. He is usually involved in large-scale human research, especially on the weight problems of adolescents, whose habits he investigates in schools and summer camps. He has been active in the Boston poverty program and has advised the World Health Organization and the Food and Agriculture Organization. He has helped the federal space program work out the dietary needs of astronauts. He is also raising a family of five children, aged six to twenty. (All statistics in this book are given as of the time of our interviews.)

Unlike most middle-aged males, Dr. Mayer, who served as a commando officer with the Free French forces during World War II, actually enjoys physical exertion. "I have a joy in moving my body," he said.

"When I have my month's vacation and sail and play tennis five or six times a week, it's a great pleasure seeing muscles reappear. It's like being a self-inflicted Pygmalion: man reemerging out of the flab. The joy of moving should be a natural thing. I'm happy when I move well."

During the rest of the year exercise remains a nagging problem. Dr. Mayer tries to avoid elevators. He plants trees at his large, comfortably rambling old home in the country near Sudbury, Massachusetts. He tries to walk regularly, but business often interferes. Three days a week, however, he usually walks to his club for lunch (one hour both ways), and he does his best to expend maximum energy during this workout.

"I walk faster than anybody else in the street," he said. "I like it. No phones. It's the one time when I can think."

The bitter truth is, nevertheless, that Dr. Mayer, like most American men, cannot really work off much more than five hundred calories a day through exercise, and he can't even do *that* every day without neglecting what he finds infinitely more stimulating: his work. The only way out, then, is to eat moderately and selectively. Desserts are taboo ("I avoid them like the plague"). Favorite dishes like *cervelle au beurre noir* Dr. Mayer still eats, but only "once in a while." Other weaknesses he deals with in the same way.

"I'm very fond of *pâté de foie gras*," he said with a slight sigh, "but I don't believe in punishing myself. I try to replace it with some lobster, if I can."

Besides adhering to his savings programs for calories *per se*, Dr. Mayer also has become convinced that he, like almost every American, should eat less fat, especially animal fat. This conviction did not hit him overnight; far from it. It began slowly, roughly fifteen years ago, when important experimental findings on the effects of fat on the human body first became known in the scientific community. Almost every year since then, new evidence was developed, and Dr. Mayer took further personal measures, more or less to take into account what he considered to be the meaning of the new research.

He began by almost completely eliminating milk, except occasionally in coffee. "I like American milk," he said, "but I cut down progressively. I certainly don't need the butterfat. It only gives me riboflavin and calcium, and I make sure I get that from fish, fruit and vegetables. I don't think milk is bad for me. I'd just rather have a good glass of wine."

Then, some twelve years or more ago, he gave up butter. He claims to "despise" margarine, so he has used no table spread at all ever since, except marmalade for his breakfast toast (one slice, along with orange juice and tea).

About two years later he gave up fried eggs and had them poached or soft-boiled. Three years ago he gave up eggs almost completely. "I eat them when I'm a house guest," he said.

Then, about two years ago, Dr. Mayer began cutting down greatly on his principal (and favorite) staple: meat. "The American public thinks meat is 'low-cal,'" he said. "It isn't." The public also is not generally aware that meat contains considerable fat. "I used to be a great steak and roast man," the doctor continued, "but I've been wanting to cut down on saturated [animal] fats. It's been a progressive phenomenon with me, and it's amazing how easy it is. As I got older, my taste began to change. I don't like meat as well. I eat some ham, and I am fond of things like salami and *charcuterie* [cold cuts], but I usually have those things just for a picnic in the mountains. On the whole, I have cut down drastically on meat. Now, when I go out, I practically never *choose* meat or liver or kidneys. Fortunately, I've always liked fish. I suppose fish, bread and fruit are probably my main foods. I also eat a lot of salad with vinegar and corn oil."

Nowadays Dr. Mayer's lunches usually consist of fish (rich in polyunsaturated fats). He likes scallops and oysters, and while he consumes "lots of tuna-fish sandwiches," he also has lobster as often as he feels he can afford it. "It's got everything in my favor," he said. "It's so much work that you don't eat much."

At dinner Dr. Mayer usually eats a conventional American entrée, but less than average-sized portions. Not infrequently, however, when his wife and children have hamburger (which is always made of ground chuck, not standard supermarket hamburger meat), the doctor makes a concession to one of his most insidious weaknesses: the craving for good cheese. But he has cheese *instead* of beef, not at the same meal. "The trouble with cheese is that it always comes when you've already had too much to eat," he said. So he often makes a meal of jellied consommé, cheese, bread and fruit.

Jellied consommé, of which the doctor is exceptionally fond and which is delightfully low in calories, is also one of his major standbys as a snack. He usually has some at bedtime. Or else he may nibble on some bread and cheese, usually cottage cheese because it contains less fat than most other cheeses. Apples are another standard snack, and when Dr. Mayer finds himself the victim of particularly vicious between-meal hunger pangs, he has been known to gobble as many as three apples at a sitting. Occasionally he even likes to snack on the leftover skin of a baked potato.

The doctor uses no special diet foods or drinks except an occasional low-calorie cola and saccharin for his coffee. "I don't go around with saccharin in my pocket," he said, "but I have it in my office and at home. If I have six cups daily with sugar, that's a hundred twenty calories. If I use just a little more sugar, that's two hundred. That's six thousand calories a month, that's two pounds of fat. I'd much rather have good bread once in a while."

Dr. Mayer is that relatively rare person who does not feel calorically tempted when he is exposed to restaurant food during his fairly frequent business travels. "I eat much better at home," he said. At banquets he also has no trouble turning down food or leaving portions of large servings on his plate. ("I'm a professor of nutrition. I can afford to be rude. If I refuse food, I'm doing my job.")

If this suggests that the doctor is a practicing auto-crat—and he is—it should not suggest that he is anything but gregarious, too. He likes parties, and his normal eating and drinking habits are sufficiently moderate so he can afford to nibble on nuts and other cocktail snacks and enjoy a drink or two, even the relatively high-calorie drinks that he likes best, like daiquiris and Bacardis. He is also fond of beer, especially Guinness dark ale. The point is that he does not load up with any of these treats as a regular habit.

"I had a bottle of ale about a week ago," he told us when we saw him.

Like all the doctors' wives we met, the American-born Mrs. Mayer harbors no reservations about the soundness of her husband's ideas about food. Elizabeth Mayer, relaxed and somewhat reserved, also admits to being lucky: Her appetite is small. At forty-six, she is five feet six and a half inches tall and weighs 119 pounds. About fifteen years ago she weighed 115 pounds. Her tastes are simpler than her husband's. She is not overly enthusiastic about cooking, and the business of shopping in accordance with the Doctors' Diet comes naturally to her.

Her children eat butter, but two pounds for seven people lasts comfortably for the whole week. Mayonnaise? Mrs. Mayer buys perhaps two jars a year. Cookies? "Not very often. They get stale around this house." Potato chips? "Only for picnics." Commercially baked desserts? "We had four raspberry turnovers here lately; they took a week to eat up." But there are peaches and apples always on the table, and plenty of raw carrots, sliced cucumbers and apple juice in the refrigerator.

"I eat the way the children do, but less," Mrs. Mayer reported. And the youngsters "eat anything as long as it's steak." The two older sons went through what their father calls "a puppy-fat stage," but they outgrew it normally. The seventeen-year-old daughter is "convinced she has a weight problem, but she doesn't." She is five feet four and weighs 115 pounds. The doctor does not make a point of discussing diet problems at home ("We speak far, far less about food than most people"), although he has firmly and successfully urged all his youngsters to be active in sports. "They win a lot of track events," he said with considerable pride.

Oftentimes a pattern emerges most clearly from a single undramatic illustration, and perhaps the Mayer family's way of eating comes best into focus in their attitude toward bacon. Two of the five children don't like it and don't eat it. Three do like it and have two or three strips fairly frequently. When they do, Mrs. Mayer always has one strip. The doctor, on the other hand, hasn't touched bacon in years.

It doesn't seem to bother him. None of his dietary self-denials do; principally—or so we have become convinced—this is because his skeptical researcher's mind has accepted that the recent medical findings on eating and exercise are on the right track and that they apply to him personally as a middle-aged, heart-disease-prone male. We also believe it to be significant that Dr. Mayer possesses an intellectual facility that is surprisingly uncommon: the ability not only to look and plan ahead but also to see himself actually functioning within the context of the long-range future—a very distant time that most people can't (or don't care to) visualize and therefore don't usually bother to provide for. It is this capacity, we think, that caused the doctor to tell us: "Everybody always claims they don't want to live forever. I do—if I can be fit. There are more rewarding things even than *pâté de foie gras*. I want to be around and know what's going to happen."

3

DR. STARE : *Swallowing His Own Medicine*

We can't prove it, of course, but it's entirely conceivable that no other American thinks and talks more about food than Dr. Fredrick Stare. If our private theory is correct, there would be perfectly sensible professional as well as personal justifications for it. As chairman of his specialty's most prestigious teaching center in the United States, the Department of Nutrition at the Harvard University School of Public Health, Dr. Stare is practically required to be a vociferous propagandist for sound diet habits. And as one of the unfortunates who craves food more than many of his colleagues, he must marshal the most meticulous attention to his own habits so he cannot ever be accused of not practicing what he preaches with such fervor.

In fact, Dr. Stare is so widely known for his speeches, books, newspaper columns, radio broadcasts, and for his omnipresence wherever diet is a serious subject of discussion, that we venture the following prediction: If Fred Stare ever gains weight visibly, the nation's nutritionists will feel as deserted as the Seven Dwarfs without Snow White.

Judging by Dr. Stare's past record and his current eating and drinking habits, this emergency is unlikely to occur.

The first thing you notice when you meet Dr. Stare, who is fifty-six and five feet ten inches tall, is his almost dazzlingly boyish appearance. His hair is curly and only beginning to gray. His cheeks are lean and pink. His voice crackles like that of an infantry lieutenant just out of Officers' Candidate School, and his waistline, too, makes you think of fellows in their twenties who run obstacle courses before breakfast. Fred Stare never walks; he strides at a near-run. Nor does he sit; he merely gets coiled up, and only very temporarily.

Dr. Stare works harder than any other man we

know to maintain his youthful appearance and the vibrant health that must support it. His motivation is made of unusually strong stuff. Not only does he believe in the importance of good nutrition with all the fervor of a convert ever ready to testify for his religion. There are personal factors: His first wife, who was always somewhat overweight, died of heart disease at forty-two; and since one of his key functions at Harvard is fund-raising among hardheaded (and often soft-bellied) businessmen, he knows his figure is under constant skeptical scrutiny.

"When I'm eating out," the doctor reported, "people always wait and say, 'I want to see what you order.'"

Unfortunately, Dr. Stare's own body cooperates only with reluctance. "I enjoy eating," the doctor said. "I even like black, crispy, crunchy fat."

His second wife, Helen (five feet five and a half, 130 pounds), an attractive, blonde, former newspaper reporter who is in her forties, told him while we were visiting: "You would put away anything I'd put in front of you."

Dr. Stare only smiled.

Despite his weakness for food (or perhaps because he recognizes it so well), the doctor has weighed no less than 148 and no more than 152 pounds for more than twenty-five years. Whenever he hits 152, he cuts down a little. He weighs himself at home twice a month, always on a Sunday morning before breakfast, and also whenever he visits his clubs, the Harvard in New York and the Cosmos in Washington, where a record is kept of his weight. "I don't count calories," he told us. "No one does that I know of. The way to count calories is to get on the scale."

In his appointment book the doctor also records the weight of his three children, aged fourteen to twenty-seven, but not his wife's. "She doesn't like for me to keep a record," even this determined doctor admitted. "It's not worth an argument."

We had learned beforehand of Dr. Stare's punctilious ways, and we also knew that he was considerably less inclined than most doctors to maintain a caloric double standard for the benefit of guests who live less resolutely than he. We were therefore pleased and more than slightly titillated to receive an invitation to be weekend house guests of the Stares on their fifty-acre farm outside Wellesley, Massachusetts.

Let's say it right away. The Stares are model hosts. Their home runs like an exquisite Swiss watch. Their house is quietly elegant on the inside and braced for an active life on the outside (there are four donkeys for daughter Mary, fourteen, and her friends, and the woods are overrun with rhododendrons planted by the doctor himself). No, we didn't starve, either. At the same time, the visit was a calorically interesting experience, which is undoubtedly exactly what Fred Stare had had in mind.

On Saturday night there was a dinner party. Besides ourselves, there were Dr. Stare's Harvard colleagues, Dr. Jean Mayer and his wife, and our friend Tom Winship, managing editor of the Boston *Globe,* and his wife. The cocktail hour was relaxed. No dietary restrictions were noticeable, although the principal hors d'oeuvre, along with the usual nuts, was a crunchy delicacy that turned out to be pickled eggplant.

Dinner was delicious. We had fish poached in wine, mushrooms, carrots, tossed salad, and excellent white wine served in rather small glasses. There was no bread or butter. There was also no talk of food: The company was stimulating, and we were all too busy talking about other things. We knew that Dr. Stare holds forceful views on the subject of "seconds" ("I *never* push them"), and so we were frankly curious how this problem would be circumnavigated in his own home on such an obviously festive occasion. In the interests of truthful diet reporting, then, we are compelled to pass along the word that Dr. Stare has found a way to eliminate the entire problem effectively. When the silver platters were passed for the second time, the platters were nicely visible; the food was not. We gluttons helped ourselves to a little more of everything, naturally. Very little. Luckily, most of the others at the table didn't.

There was sherbet for dessert, and we noticed that our host had a scoop like everybody else.

The next morning Mrs. Stare and the Wydens had scrambled eggs and very well-done sausage, but Dr. Stare just mixed himself several kinds of dry cereal in a bowl and had the mélange with some regular milk ("I'm not a skim-milk devotee; it's almost like putting water on cereal").

Later the doctor told us that he really does not enjoy this sort of self-denial. "It would have been most pleasant to have had a couple of sausages and eggs for breakfast. And last night that dessert tasted mighty good to me." Although Mrs. Stare enjoys baking an occasional cake, the Stares almost never have desserts unless there are guests.

While Dr. Stare has quite evidently always been master of his appetite, we found it significant that this physician, whose role as an educator is perhaps more public than that of any of the other experts we interviewed, has made some fairly drastic changes in his habits in recent years.

About seven or eight years ago he stopped eating table spreads.

About six years ago he stopped putting sugar on his cereal.

Also about six years ago he began making a conscious switch from meat to fish whenever possible. Mrs. Stare does not happen to like fish very much, so the doctor usually has it for lunch or on other occasions when he eats out, which is quite often.

About four years ago he almost stopped eating any egg yolks, even in salad. He does have whole eggs once or twice a month, usually when he is traveling and having breakfast on planes.

The doctor has also cut down on orange juice (he has two or three ounces now, instead of six or seven); pork ("I've never cared too much for it"), including sausages and bacon; butter and margarine in baked potatoes, which he is fond of ("I used damned little"); and visible fat on meat ("I'm definitely more conscientious about cutting off fat").

He has increased his consumption of soup ("I usually have a generous bowlful with a handful of crackers") and poultry, which he says he now prefers to meat.

Some of the switches and restrictions are designed to cut down on cholesterol (especially the changes in fish and egg consumption), but most of them (even the changes in orange juice and sugar) help the doctor pare down his routine consumption of calories —and for a very specific reason. As the years went by, he found that he drank a little more than before. He likes to linger over a stiff three-ounce Scotch before dinner and always has a highball or two around 10 P.M.

"I find it restful and relaxing," he said. "But I have to save room for it."

Dr. Stare is a small-town Midwesterner (he hails from Columbus, Wisconsin), and waste is abhorrent to him. At the same time, one of his chronic lectures, delivered to anyone who will listen, concerns "that dreadful, ridiculous habit of 'clean up your plate!' " The doctor deals with this apparent conflict by never putting much on his plate in the first place. Not long ago, when he lunched with a group of businessmen, he ordered nothing but a bowl of vichyssoise ("They were very embarrassed," he reported with unconcealed delight). We asked him about another of his business lunches, and he said, "I had half a sandwich."

When he goes to a restaurant, he attempts to persuade the waiters to cooperate with his habits. "Bring me a smallish portion," he likes to say, "and please don't cover it up with a sauce."

Such efforts to keep his plate half-vacant do not always work. When they don't, Dr. Stare is likely to get upset. "Look at all this food," he says. "Revolting!"

Nevertheless, he does admit to hunger pangs, and he does nibble between meals. After a fashion. When he gets "quite hungry" in the afternoon—and he always does—he usually has just a cup of coffee. At home he snacks a lot on fruit. He is fond of Liederkranz and crackers, but usually has so little of the cheese that Mrs. Stare winds up throwing away even much of a small package. The doctor considers potato chips a formidable weakness, and often has them for a bedtime snack, but he does not park himself in front of a bag of chips. "I have half a dozen," he said, "and only if my wife *brings* them."

In fact, one of the doctor's more effective measures for dealing with temptation is simply a conscious effort to stay out of the kitchen.

Within the past six or seven years Dr. Stare has also given "very definite renewed emphasis" to the importance of getting some physical exercise regularly. His is the standard lament centering on the necessarily sedentary nature of his work. He phrased the problem succinctly: "When I'm in Boston, I'm more or less paid to sit." Yet he has found techniques for escaping his executive chair often enough to help him maintain his enviable condition. It simply requires determination plus not too much concern about exhibiting some mildly unconventional habits in public.

In his modern office building he never uses the elevator. When he goes downtown for a twice-a-week radio show about the blessings of good nutrition, he takes the subway only part of the way and "walks" the rest, always in his own rather special manner. ("I do it even if I'm pressed for time, and I damned near *run*.") The doctor and his wife started playing tennis four years ago. ("It's a good opportunity to be together.") In winter they play twice a week on inside courts, in summer three times a week. During the winter months Dr. Stare also takes time out to play squash twice a week.

During his frequent business trips the doctor makes a special point of seeking out ways to move his body as vigorously as he possibly can. "I always look for distances to get in a fast ten-minute walk," he said, and what Dr. Stare calls fast might seem like track training speed to most Americans. Arriving at Kennedy Airport in New York, he usually takes a taxi as far as 59th Street and Fifth Avenue and then scampers down Fifth Avenue to 44th Street to the Harvard Club at a pace that would seem inconsistent with Harvard dignity. On his way to business appointments he usually takes the subway but gets off at an earlier stop than necessary and then again breaks into his near-trot.

Mrs. Stare knows that there is a less urgent medical need for women to seek physical exertion, and she is grateful. She enjoys her family tennis sessions and often parks her car a few blocks away from her destination in order to create an opportunity for a walk. "But I don't like exercise for the sake of exercise," she said.

Dietary restrictions are something else again. Helen Stare is acutely conscious of her wifely role in keeping her husband healthy. "It really is up to any woman to determine what her husband is going to be," she said. "If I wanted to make my husband obese, I could do it sneakily. For instance, he loves scallops made with lots of butter and cream so they're nice and crunchy. But we have practically no butter in the house. I use less than a pound a week for four people."

Mrs. Stare never, but never, fixes any fried food. She uses very little salt, because Dr. Stare, like a few other doctors we interviewed, has become convinced that excessive salt consumption may encourage hypertension and water retention. Mrs. Stare cooks with margarine and vegetable oils and never uses as much fat as recommended in cookbook recipes ("not even with scallops"). Steak is served only once every three weeks or even less often in the Stare household, and Helen Stare almost always buys a relatively low-priced, low-fat cut, such as London broil ("I feel sinful when I get a good steak"). Meat loaf, too, is on the dinner menu only about once every three weeks. Hamburger is considered a treat and is always made of ground round or chuck. Standard dishes include lean roast beef, pot roast, chicken, chicken livers, ham and fish.

The Stares are alert to the fact that weight can easily be influenced by emotional factors. Both of the doctor's sons put on pounds after the death of their mother, and Dr. Stare finds he must make a particular effort not to eat extra food when he gets upset for any reason. However, even this unusually zealous educator never lectured his children about food.

"I've tried to set good food habits by good example," he said. "We've always served the children a good variety of foods. We give them relatively small portions and would rather have them come back for 'thirds' than give them too much in the first place. We've always tried to keep candy out of the house. When it's around, I might eat it, too. Desserts aren't much trouble. They're just not there. Just a couple of times a week there may be a dish of ice cream."

Helen Stare confirmed: "Fred never told me what

to do except, 'All I ask is that you don't put too much butter on things.' "

Daughter Mary, fourteen, did not seem unhappy about the caloric state of affairs at home, although she did register a mild protest about her father's substitute for candy. "Instead, he gives us *books*," she said, feigning disgust. On the other hand, Mary has never had a weight problem, and we doubt that she ever will.

4

THE ALEXANDERS : *Two Experts in the Family*

What happens in a family when husband and wife both qualify as diet experts? Do they compete with each other in experimenting with ever-new scientific methods for weight management? Do they talk about diets all the time? Do they disagree frequently, as doctors (or, for that matter, husbands and wives) tend to do? We came for the answers to the big, comfortable old Boston home of Dr. and Mrs. Benjamin Alexander. At the time of our visit he was an associate professor at the Harvard School of Medicine, a specialist in hematology (disease of the blood) and practiced at Beth Israel Hospital. His research has been in the field of blood clotting. He now is clinical professor of medicine at Cornell University Medical School. Marie Alexander, who used to head the food clinic at Beth Israel, still works as a research associate for Dr. Stare at Harvard and also helps him write his newspaper column on nutrition problems, even though she and her husband now live in New York. Both the Alexanders are in their fifties. Their children are twenty-three, twenty-one and seventeen.

The answers to our questions turned out to be agreeably unspectacular. Both husband and wife have made their own adjustments so they can control their respective weight problems, and they have done this without much advice or argument passing back and forth. Each has applied the recent medical findings to his own appetite and health problems. Each eats and exercises accordingly. In Mrs. Alexander's case, few changes were necessary. In her husband's case, the changes were drastic.

Marie Alexander happens to be one of the lucky ones. Quiet, thin-faced and bespectacled, she measures five feet six inches, and her weight has remained steady at 140 pounds since college. "I'm careful," she said. "I find it easy to gain two or three pounds when I'm on vacation." Clearly, however, her appetite is not a constant nagging problem.

She still has eggs for breakfast three or four mornings a week, but they are rarely fried now ("We fry less and less"). Her typical lunch is a cheese sandwich on rye bread (with margarine, not butter), perhaps a tomato, a piece of fruit, a glass of regular milk or a cup of coffee with saccharin (the family switched from sugar six years ago). If Mrs. Alexander has hunger pangs in midafternoon, she may have a plain cookie or two, but usually she was too busy getting her daily exercise: cleaning her eight-room house and running up and down between the upstairs floors and the laundry in the basement. In Boston she also often walked to and from work, a distance of one and a quarter miles, but conceded that "it's kind of sporadic."

The Alexanders used to have a "sociable hour" over a drink before dinner, but they are not overly fond of alcohol and did not miss their cocktails when they decided to abandon them. Wine is served at dinner once every two or four weeks, and there are no bedtime snacks ("It's a poor idea"). There are "practically never" any snack foods like potato chips or pretzels in the house. The evening meal, however, is conventional.

You won't find high-fat foods like French fried potatoes on this dinner table, and about three years ago Mrs. Alexander started cooking with margarine just about exclusively (she buys butter a quarter of a pound at a time). Cole slaw and potato salad are unheard of, and all frying has been done in a Teflon pan for more than five years. But when the Alexanders have steak, it is a tender cut of top quality, and desserts are almost always served, including chocolate pie and sweet rolls, though rarely ice cream or other high-fat dairy foods. There is fish once or twice a week, chicken and veal usually once a week, and very little talk about food at any time.

For Ben Alexander, weight management has meant a considerable and continuing effort, but it has paid off nicely: At six feet, he weighs 160 pounds, the same as five years before, and this compares with 154 pounds when he was in college. Unfortunately, he gets hungrier than his wife and must watch himself carefully.

"I'm diet-conscious," he said. "I have to work at it constantly." He also claimed, "I'm not a very strongly disciplined person," although it would be rather difficult to document this with his daily routine.

Dr. Alexander gave up just about all visible eggs about nine years ago, although he will occasionally have half an egg in a salad. He used to eat two eggs

for breakfast, but he came to believe that the cholesterol in eggs is somehow more efficiently absorbed into
the bloodstream than the cholesterol contained in
other foods. Seven years ago he gave up putting butter
or margarine on his breakfast toast. Instead, he lines
up five or six kinds of jam and picks one that he
hasn't used for a few days. He gave up milk (except
in coffee) at the age of 40, but still enjoys cheese,
although he "emphasizes" cottage cheese as much as
possible.

"I feel all dairy fats are bad for me," he said. He
also strips the skin from chicken because it absorbs
a lot of fat, and when he cuts off steak he invariably
makes certain that he trims a little meat, too, so
that not one bit of avoidable fat will enter his system.

Dr. Alexander's most notable recent health measure
has been to add more exercise to his working day.
"On the basis of my reading I feel it's important,"
he said. "I also feel better now."

He begins by raising each leg alternately twenty-
four times at 7 A.M. while he is still in bed. He then
does twelve or fourteen push-ups. "There are many
days when I don't feel like doing it," he said, "and
I always have a good excuse, like 'I have an early committee meeting.' But I have a strong motivation. Exercise is good for everybody's bones, and I have a
feeling, based on my own research, that it improves

the blood." Some years ago he tried playing golf, but
when he discovered that he did not care for the game,
he started walking around the hospital's city block a
few times during his lunch hour. Three years ago,
however, he found he simply did not have the time
and gave it up.

Now he walks to and from work, one mile each
way, "even in a blizzard, but not in the rain." At
work he looks for excuses not to pick up a phone and
walks instead. Another rule: "I never take an elevator
if I can help it." He added: "My office is on the
third floor, and I have taken four flights from time
to time, fast, as a special push. It's a conscious, deliberate effort." Six months before our visit, the
doctor had added still another daily "push": On his
way back from the office around 6:15 P.M. he takes
the last four hundred yards through the park at a
run, juggling his briefcase as best he can.

When the Alexanders have guests, on the other
hand, all signs of any dietary regimen disappear. "I
like to feel like a hostess, not like a nutritionist. We
even *urge* everbody to have seconds." The Alexander
children, too, have not been exposed to special parental lectures on eating and exercise, although it is
obvious that they have absorbed nutritional good
sense around the house.

"At exam time my eating goes to pot," said Judy,

a Radcliffe senior who measures five feet eight, weighs 136 pounds, and admits to having reached 141 from time to time. "But we all know we shouldn't use too much milk, for example. Most of my friends have no idea about these things. They won't eat a piece of bread, but they'll eat five pieces of fruit instead, which is much more fattening."

Marie Alexander reported that she could not remember having ever cracked down hard on their children's eating habits ("It wouldn't have done any good") even though there were times when seventeen-year-old Robert, for instance, might have deserved it. Somehow he did not remain a problem. His mother told us, "When I offer him an extra now, he feels it's poison."

5

DR. STAMLER : *Gluttony Under Control*

"I never do anything in moderation," said Dr. Jeremiah Stamler, the gregarious, beetle-browed, little whirling dervish who is director of the Division of Adult Health and Aging and head of the Heart Disease Control Section of the Chicago Board of Health. As far as his eating is concerned, the doctor had his tense wrong. It is true that he did not eat with moderation for most of his life. A high-school cartoon portrayed him with a formidable paunch. In his later years he was so fond of meat that friends, watching him tuck it away, used to needle him by asking whether he was a member of the meat packer's union. By the mid-1950's, the doctor weighed 165 pounds, which is a little hefty for a man who is only five feet four inches tall. But then something happened. Now, at forty-seven, he is a svelte 143 pounds. His blood cholesterol level is still rather high at 260 (he would like it to be 215), but Dr. Stamler is convinced he is no longer anywhere near as likely a candidate for a heart attack as he was some years ago.

What happened?

Well, Dr. Stamler's personality did not change. He still says, with the boyish verve that is his trademark, "I have to struggle all the time. I *love* to eat." He still craves (and enjoys) beer, bagels and very spicy foods ("I don't have exquisite taste"), and he can still gobble a basketful of breadsticks. Nevertheless, what happened was nothing more nor less than a total reorientation of the doctor's eating habits. He simply read and analyzed the scientific findings as they became available in the medical journals, and decided it would be foolish not to apply them promptly to himself and his family. He not only cut down drastically on his total intake of calories. He also greatly increased his exercise. He became one of the nation's most outspoken advocates of a diet that is not only low in all fats but particularly low in animal fats.

And when the government's nationwide diet-heart study began, the doctor became its principal administrator for the Chicago area.

Until the mid-1950's Dr. Stamler had hardly ever weighed himself. Now he steps on the scale five days a week. Bacon, eggs and rich cheeses were staples in his daily diet; now he has eggs just once a month, bacon (very well done) less than once a month, and he has switched to special cheese spreads containing only four percent fat. He has learned to cope with his immoderate appetite partly by applying self-discipline (which was easier to muster because of his conviction that he was practicing sound preventive medicine on himself and his family) and partly by teaching himself to make substitutions for certain foods.

"It's not so much a question of sacrifice," he insisted. "It's a matter of changing your taste."

With characteristic enthusiasm Dr. Stamler maintains that fundamental taste changes are not only relatively easy to accomplish, once you put your mind to it; he also claims that newly acquired tastes can actually wipe away old ones. For example, the doctor used to drink eight cups of coffee a day with milk and two spoonfuls of sugar each. Then he began to calculate that he was ingesting three hundred calories a day via the coffee route alone. "That's a lot of calories!" he exclaimed. "So then I started using saccharin. I liked coffee sweet. At a certain point some years ago I asked myself, 'Why take a chemical all my life?' I stopped using it. For a week coffee tasted funny. Now I *hate* sweet coffee. It tastes terrible! I don't see how people can drink it."

The doctor's wife, Rose, a sociologist who works in her husband's office and develops community programs for the prevention of chronic diseases, reports that she experienced a similar reaction to the withdrawal of fats. "After a few years the taste for fatty foods just becomes eliminated," she said. "Duck used to be my favorite food. Now it gives me indigestion."

Fortunately, Dr. Stamler is so fond of all bread and rolls that he enjoys them dry (he gave up table spreads years ago). This enables him to start the morning with a "sizable chunk" of watermelon or other fresh fruit, two freshly heated rolls and a plain tomato. If he has lunch in the office, it is likely to be a tuna-fish sandwich or a chicken or turkey sandwich with mayonnaise on the side. Lunch with friends and associates outside the office could be a problem for Dr. Stamler, who best enjoys eating when he is in good company. He either has a sandwich or a shrimp or tuna-fish salad bowl ("I take the yolk out of the sliced eggs; it's poison") or a "huge" tureen of soup plus a pasta dish with meat sauce. The little breadsticks in his favorite Italian restaurants have become his dessert, "and I'll have ten instead of forty," along with coffee.

During the day the doctor makes a point of snacking on nothing except fruit. ("I *love* fruit. I can eat as much as two pounds a day, and that gets to be a real carbohydrate problem.")

For dinner at home there is either a highball *or* wine, never both. Once or twice a week there is chicken, usually rotisserie-broiled or perhaps dressed up as chicken cacciatore. Once a week there is a shrimp dish, either fried in vegetable oil or boiled with rice. The doctor eats meat no more than a total of five times a week, and he is delighted that his official position has helped to give him access to a special source of particularly lean cuts.

Because of his professional activities, Dr. Stamler often has dinner away from home, sometimes several times a week. If he must go to a cocktail party first, he tries to limit himself to one highball or one beer, and he favors the hors d'oeuvres made of fish. Banquets are a time for self-restraint. "I went to a dinner last night," he said, "and had about half the portion of roast beef, no potatoes, all the vegetable, I enjoyed the roll dry, and I had one spoonful of the ice cream." Passing up the dessert was still somewhat painful, the doctor confessed.

"I used to eat a lot of ice cream," he said "I *love* ice cream!"

Like so many of our interviewees, Dr. Stamler has a distinct eating problem in the evening, usually toward midnight. This is a time when his long-established tastes are hard to hide, and a mere nibble on some nuts does not interest him at all. He may have a highball and a sandwich of water-packed tuna, or two bagels with sliced tomatoes, or a piece of thin-sliced pumpernickel with low-fat cheese, or pressed smoked thin-sliced meats such as turkey or beef, which are extremely low in fat.

"If I'm trying to control my weight, I eliminate the alcohol," he reported. "And if I'm really struggling, then I have just half a grapefruit before going to bed. But I *hate* that."

There is only one reason why the doctor never had an even greater weight problem than he had some years ago, and it is perfectly apparent even after you have only seen him operate in his office for a few minutes. Among all the many restless, hyper-energetic doctors we met, Dr. Stamler manages to stand out. In his cluttered office he seems all but airborne: darting up and down, ducking out the door and back again, conducting conversations with assistants, doing paper work and talking on the telephone somehow at the same time. Yet there is always a lot more energy to spare.

"Nothing makes me feel better than a good swim, a good workout," he said.

Every morning he starts out with calisthenics—only five minutes' worth (mostly leg-raising), but at a very rapid pace, and he always makes sure to work up a real sweat. His office at the Chicago Board of Health is on the fourth floor, and he always walks up unless he is heavily loaded down with bundles. At Northwestern University he holds a regular clinic, which is on the third floor. He always walks up there, too. And he makes it a point almost never to go to meetings of the Chicago Heart Association (one mile each way from his own office) except on foot.

Five years ago Dr. Stamler bought a stationary exercising bicycle for his home. He finds this device "very boring," but nevertheless brings himself to use it two or three times a week. More recently he purchased a real bicycle for use in the summer and has been using it three or four times a week, each time for a quarter to half an hour. Three times a week, for more than ten years now, Dr. Stamler has been swimming at his neighborhood "Y"—usually between 8 and 9 P.M.—and when he travels, he always takes along his swimming trunks and stays at a hotel with a pool or with a "Y" nearby.

"When I don't get exercise, I get restive," he said. "It's a form of relief of tension."

Mrs. Stamler, who is considerably more relaxed than her husband, follows no large-scale program of organized exercise, but her pattern of eating is much like his. At forty-one, she measures five feet seven and a half inches, weighs 130 pounds and normally does not have much trouble controlling her weight. Her breakfast is the same as the doctor's. Her lunch mainstay is a sandwich, but she is more relaxed about consuming animal fats than Dr. Stamler is; occasionally she will have a liverwurst or egg or cheese sandwich. At home, however, she supports the doctor's convictions even to the extent of making her own popcorn in order to be able to prepare it with vegetable oil. At her cocktail parties, too, she serves unsaturated foods. Her hors d'oeuvres are mostly of the fish variety (shrimp, sardines, anchovy paste), served with crackers. Her usual cookies are ginger snaps.

"I never buy pie," Mrs. Stamler said. "Half a dozen times a year or so I make my own, and about three times a year I buy a pineapple cheese cake. But I'm the only one who eats it."

The Stamlers' sixteen-year-old son, Paul, does not happen to be one of those nonfinicky young eaters whom we met in many doctors' families. "He doesn't like steak or fish, and he doesn't know what vegetables are," said his mother. "We have a lot of hamburger and kind of fill up on salads, beans, mushrooms, green peppers, pimentos and things like that. Paul will eat chocolate cake when he's out, but we don't make a big deal of it. Sometimes he's a little overweight, but he eats a gigantic amount of peanut butter a week."

The Stamlers are relaxed about it: "After the third sandwich in two hours, we'll say, 'Isn't that enough?' "

The Stamlers, then, *are* preoccupied with food and have very distinctive tastes. Yet they are counteracting the great American problem of fat intake with some success, and their larder is usually well-filled ("There's not a feeling of austerity in the house"). Beyond that, there is an attitude of enthusiasm about diets, a sense of continuous curiosity about new diet research and useful findings still to come.

Characteristically, one of the showpieces in Dr. Stamler's office is a cartoon of two men talking. The caption says, "The trouble is all the important discoveries have already been made."

The men in the cartoon are cavemen.

6

DR. WHITE : *Staying Trim Under Pressure*

We don't know of anyone in America who is more embarrassingly on the spot every time he sits down to eat than Dr. Philip L. White of Chicago. As director of the Department of Foods and Nutrition of the American Medical Association, he is a central source of guidance on nutrition matters for a sizable segment of the medical profession, the food industry (which is, after all, the nation's largest business) and the many audiences—professional, academic and just plain public—that Dr. White is continually asked to address so that they may get the latest word about staying healthy by eating "right."

As we have seen, the "right" way to eat is mostly a matter of taste, habit, self-discipline, body demands and an individual's own interpretation of recent medical findings. Reconciling these elements is not always simple. Consciously or otherwise, however, Dr. White must also consider some others as he picks up his own knife and fork. He is an exceptionally well-informed man; new developments in nutrition usually come to his attention at once. Yet he learned long ago that "breakthroughs" in his field almost invariably turn out, on close inspection, to be disappointments or worse. As the A.M.A.'s spokesman on nutrition, he must further keep in mind that his bosses tend to be conservative and friendly toward industry, but that they cannot afford to be (and rarely are) unreceptive to change dictated by scientific progress. Finally, he can never be unaware that his own well-watched statements and habits have serious economic implications.

We'd hate to be in Dr. White's shoes (or in the collective shoes of the dairy industry). To cite a hypothetical example: If Phil White were to turn down a dish of ice cream at a medical banquet and announce loudly, "Thank you, but I never touch it anymore!" the ensuing pressures and recriminations would be memorable.

As it happens, Dr. White, who is forty-four and was trained at Harvard, is a man of conscience and diplomacy. To meet this somewhat pale, bespectacled scientist and to listen to his precision-tooled speech is to realize at once that this is not someone who is given to acting out foolish impulses, if he has any. But to watch him smoke cigarette after cigarette is to know that here is a man who is under constant pressure and that he is feeling it all the time. In point of fact, Dr. White smokes two and a half packs of cigarettes a day. Two years ago he tried seriously to stop smoking, but the moratorium lasted only two weeks. He frankly regards cigarettes as "pacifiers" and has even been known to concede that they fill appetite-depressing functions for him as well. Anyway, breaking the smoking habit turned out to be impossible for this well-disciplined man.

"I found my work output went down," he said. "Instead of thinking about what I was doing, I was thinking, 'when can I have a cigarette?' "

Fortunately, the changes that Dr. White decided to make in his eating habits came easier to him. The doctor weighs himself only once every six weeks, but he is one of those meticulous self-observers who can tell when his stomach is expanding ever so slightly (he always shaves before putting on a shirt or undershirt) or when his belt comes under a little extra pressure. At the time of our interview he weighed 158 pounds (his height is five feet ten and a half inches), and this figure reflects the one important food change that Dr. White has made: He eats less than he once did.

"I don't intend to disappear," he said, but he admits that he has been influenced by recent findings that it is medically desirable, especially for sedentary middle-aged males, to weigh even less than the "ideal" weights suggested by the tables distributed by insurance companies. Thus, Dr. White weighed 162 pounds five years previously. Ten years before that he weighed 165. When we talked with him he was struggling to get down to 155.

Dr. White stopped using sugar in his coffee more than ten years ago. Shortly afterward he started drinking some skim milk every day, although at home he still uses the regular kind. He has not changed his egg consumption (four to six a week, which is moderate), but about six years ago he cut down from two slices of breakfast toast to one slice. Then he made a drastic change in his lunches, much like other experts in our survey: Instead of ordering a "normal" meat-and-potato type of meal, he confined himself to soup, a sandwich and skim milk.

Dr. White and his family have not changed their fish, meat or butter consumption in accordance with the latest theories about animal fats, but we were not exactly startled to discover that they have all along been almost as careful about high-fat foods as most of the doctors who say they feel strongly about it. The Whites have steak, for instance, about only once every two weeks in the summertime and once every three weeks during the rest of the year. They serve French fried potatoes, but only "maybe once every month or two." They do not often have dessert, and then almost never anything richer than ice cream —in modest portions and not more than three times a week. They never buy commercially baked cakes or pies. They have always used margarine ("for cost reasons"), and while Dr. White likes to be served three slices of bacon at a time, it turns out that he never has bacon more than once a week.

The Whites have hot dogs once every two or three weeks. They use the relatively low-fat ground chuck or round for hamburger (usually twice a week). Do they use care in removing fat from meat? Indeed they do. "I never really cared for fat on steak and roasts," said Dr. White. They use any salad dressings that they may hanker for, including Roquefort, but they don't use overly much of it. Dr. White will even eat butter occasionally with his restaurant meals, but he uses what he calls "reasonable caution," which means that he takes very, very little.

On the other hand, he makes generous use of that popular appetite-depressant: soup. "We've always been soup eaters," said Dr. White, and he was not talking about thick soups but the clear variety that, as all doctors know, contains vast amounts of well-seasoned but gloriously calorie-free water.

Dr. White, like many of his colleagues, prefers to drink, rather than eat, his bedtime snack. He nibbles on some potato chips or nuts "every couple of weeks maybe," but normally he has only a bourbon-and-water highball, which serves him as a "sleeping elixir." The doctor also likes beer, but he is hardly the picture of a typical expansive beer drinker. How often does he drink beer? "Occasionally." Weekends? "Yes, but not every weekend." There was, he said, one can of beer in the refrigerator right now, but it might remain there for quite a while.

While Dr. White does not admit feeling guilty about it, he still does not get a great deal more exercise than most white-collar Americans. Together with his wife, he tried the famous Canadian Air Force exercises, but they kept at it for only a little over two months. Dr. White avoids elevators when he has to go up and down one or two flights, but he rarely walks three. He walks between the railroad station and his home in suburban Wilmette, and he always marches "at a good clip," but it's only a distance of four blocks each way. From the city station to his A.M.A. office in downtown Chicago the distance is seventeen blocks, and Dr. White does make that round-trip walk except when the weather is very bad, which is all too often in Chicago. Also, he actively seeks out walking errands around the vast A.M.A. office building, and he has found that extracurricular activities don't have to be sports to produce a weight-reducing effect.

Dr. White happens to be an active singer in a church group, and found that on at least one pre-holiday occasion, when he was rehearsing nightly from 7 P.M. to midnight, his weight dropped from 162 to 154 pounds, simply as a result of all the extra hard work during the extra hours.

The true "secret" of Dr. White's diet, of course, is his ability to get along on relatively modest portions. Helping him to avoid excesses is another diet expert who is stationed right in his own kitchen: his wife, Hilda, who also holds a Ph.D. degree in nutrition and is an associate professor at Northwestern University. Mrs. White, who is five feet five and a half inches tall, weighs 140 pounds. In recent years her weight has fluctuated between 135 and 142. Like her husband, she smokes a great deal (two packs a day) and feels guilty about it ("It's a habit I'd like not to have"). She eats very much as her husband does. Her typical restaurant lunch is a sandwich and a small salad or else a casserole dish, a vegetable, a muffin and skim milk.

Mrs. White admits she sometimes gets hungry enough to feel "woozy" around 4 P.M., and she then helps herself to some skim milk or an apple, but she does not normally eat between meals. It's at dinnertime when her careful shopping and food-serving habits really pay off, not only for her own figure but for her entire family.

There is no bread or butter on the Whites' dinner table. A roast is likely to be of the rolled boneless rump variety, and three or four pounds of it make an ample meal for the doctor, his wife and their two children (Chuck, ten, and Nancy, twelve)—and there are enough leftovers for some sandwiches. When Mrs. White serves chicken, as she usually does at least once a week, two or three chicken breasts and three or four legs and thighs will be enough.

According to her husband, Mrs. White enjoys "quite a reputation" among family and friends for her lasagne, her chicken chop suey and other specialties of the house. The Whites also admit that they maintain a double standard for guests. When there's company, there will be plenty of rolls and butter and desserts like ice cream pie, and Nancy may bake a rich cake. The point is that these occasions just don't arise very often, and Mrs. White does what she can to make certain that they don't.

"I make one cherry pie in the spring and one apple pie in the fall," she said. She does buy cookies for the youngsters and even relents to the extent of letting them pick out the kinds they like best.

The Whites claim no great success in educating their children to be model eaters. "I was probably as guilty as most mothers of the 'clean plate syndrome,' " said Mrs. White. The doctor said that Chuck had been getting "chubby" and that his desserts and portions were going to have to be watched more carefully. Nor did he think that either of his youngsters was getting enough exercise; he had long ago issued orders that they would have to walk to school or ride their bikes "unless it's really raining hard." On the credit side, however, he reported that neither youngster has turned into a picky eater and that there was hope they wouldn't overeat as adults simply because their parents never did.

"The example we set for them is a reasonable one," said the doctor. He was obviously pleased with his family food record, and well he might be. None of his many bosses and watchers could ask for greater tact or more efficiency.

7

DR. BRUCE TAYLOR : *An Extremist for Good Reason*

Without exception, the doctors we interviewed were convinced that Americans eat too much fat. And, again without exception, they were trying to do something for themselves and their families in order to cut down on fat, which alone supplies more than 41 percent of the calories in the average American diet. Most of the doctors seemed to think they were behaving commendably if they were able to cut down to 30 or 35 percent fat. Then, at Evanston Hospital in suburban Chicago, we encountered a physician who estimated that he was on a ten percent fat diet! Clearly, this was a dietary extremist and (since fat is what makes many foods more palatable) a fellow with a remarkably patient stomach.

The extraordinary eater in Evanston is Dr. Bruce Taylor, chairman of the hospital's pathology department and professor of pathology at Northwestern University Medical School. We had been told that the doctor was responsible for some of the more important pioneering research in dietary fats. If he was something of a food faddist, then he certainly was not an ordinary one. And if, by eating as he did, he was taking his own medicine, it was certainly worth investigating how he managed to get along.

Dr. Taylor turned out to be an easygoing, slow-spoken man of 51 with steel-gray hair and the direct, uncomplicated manner of a county agricultural agent. He is five feet eleven and a half inches tall and weighs 165 pounds (he weighs himself three or four times a week). His blood cholesterol level is 200. He has been on a very low-fat diet since the prehistoric dawn of modern diet research: 1948. At that time he had begun studying the fat deposits in the arterial wall structure of patients who had died of heart and artery disease ("I wanted to work on something that bothered a lot of people"), and after performing autopsy after autopsy, his suspicions about the probable cause-and-effect relationship between fat consumption and many of these deaths became fairly firm.

"I became convinced that you didn't have a damned thing to lose if you cut down a lot on cholesterol and on all fat intake," he recalled.

Since it is impossible to conduct continuing diet experiments with human arteries, Dr. Taylor began manipulating fats in the diets of dogs and monkeys and then checking the effects of such changes at autopsy. At the University of North Carolina he placed a group of monkeys, with an average cholesterol level of 150, on a typical American human diet. Within three months their cholesterol was up to 250. In another three months fat deposits appeared in their arteries and their cholesterol levels ranged from 250 to 400. But would people react like monkeys? To find out, Dr. Taylor tried a similar experiment on himself. For a year he lived almost exclusively on vegetables, bread and powdered skim milk; his main staple was beans ("lots and lots of beans"). When his cholesterol level was down to 187, he started eating twelve eggs a day. Within eight weeks it was up to a rather unhealthy 287.

Today, while there is no longer any doubt that cholesterol levels can be changed by diet, new research has introduced new questions about the role of cholesterol in triggering heart attacks. Other substances and mechanisms may also be involved. However important these may eventually turn out to be, Dr. Taylor is so totally convinced that fat intake must be an arch ally of our leading killer disease that he decided to take drastic personal action based on his own findings.

And drastic it certainly is. Naturally, Dr. Taylor made all the obvious changes in his diet: He stopped eating table spreads except for jam and jelly. He cut out eggs ("I eat one a year"). He switched from regular to skim milk. He quit all cheese except cottage cheese and occasional party cheese dips. He switched from ice cream to sherbet (which he has only very rarely). He gave up pork chops, peanut butter, potato chips and nuts and began drinking his coffee black.

But Dr. Taylor applies the rules with unusual vigor. He puts mostly vinegar and only very little oil on his salad ("I like it straight"). He does not care much for fish, and eats it only once or twice a month. Yet he has meat no more than once a day (because of its relatively high fat content) and makes a conscientious effort to eat only lean cuts. When he sees a chunk of egg yolk in a salad, he carefully scoops it out and puts it aside. In order to conserve calories, he also gave up potatoes and all bread except for a slice of toast in the morning with his oatmeal.

Yes, Dr. Taylor does get hunger pangs with some frequency. He is one of those doctors who rushes off to lunch at 11:30 A.M. ("I get kind of faint") and eats substantial portions of "bulky things like vegetables, watermelon, things that fill you up." Occasionally he lunches on Metrecal. He admits to nibbling occasionally on crackers and peanuts ("You've got to cheat once in a while") and still averages six to eight cups of coffee a day and three drinks of Scotch or bourbon per evening. He has no bedtime snack.

Dr. Taylor lives by himself and frequently attends dinner parties, where his diet can become something of a social problem. However, he has learned to cover up his Spartan habits. "I eat a lot of tossed salad and pickles, beets and green beans," he said. "Then my plate looks full. You slug away at that and you look like a hero."

Dr. Taylor insists that his diet changes caused him no major problem. "I used to like crisp roasted fat," he said, "but in the last few years whenever I get very fat foods sneaked into me—maybe a casserole—I get a little sick. I guess my gall bladder has been too lazy too long." He has also been able to rationalize many of his customs on the basis of personal taste preference.

"Why destroy the exquisite flavor of a nice tomato by putting blue cheese all over it?" he asked.

Like most doctors for whom substantial changes in food patterns produced few problems, Dr. Taylor was lucky in that his diet in childhood and adolescence had never been high in fats. The son of a South Dakota lumber dealer, he grew up in a home where money was a problem and such rich foods as meat and cream were relatively scarce, while vegetables were home-grown and plentiful. In many respects, therefore, his medical considerations have merely nudged him to return to the accustomed fare of his formative years.

Unlike so many of our interviewees, Dr. Taylor is anything but a supercharged type. He moves well, but not in haste, and seems so relaxed that sitting looks like his natural posture. The truth is otherwise. The doctor has long become sold on the benefits of regular exercise for healthy arteries and works at this problem as methodically as he guards his diet. He walks to work (eight blocks, round trip). He gardens. His laboratories stretch over three floors, and he makes sure he gets around frequently and always on foot. Every night around 9 or 10 P.M. he walks his beagle a couple of miles. And when he has mail to dispatch, he gets it off one letter at a time in order to manufacture an excuse to make extra trips to the mailbox.

Very few people would want to live on so rigidly restricted a diet as Dr. Taylor, even if they, too, were living alone. Indeed, a diet so low in fats is not recommended, and a lot of people would develop uncomfortable symptoms if they tried to live on it for a long time. But the assumptions of Dr. Taylor's early research are no longer mere assumptions, and among his colleagues this doctor's diet is no longer dismissed with disdain. Dr. Taylor said, "It's really refreshing after having been called a nut for so long."

8

DR. RUBIN : *The Formerly Fat Psychiatrist*

Dr. Theodore Isaac Rubin was the only psychiatrist we interviewed and, as it happened, the only doctor in our group who had ever been grossly obese: that is, at least sixty pounds overweight. Luckily, we knew in advance that he was not the kind of dour, bearded analyst who merely listens to people gravely and doesn't say much more than an occasional, slow, "Hmmm."

We surmised this about the doctor because we had read several of his ten books. Most of them are such sensitive, very contemporary fiction as *Lisa and David,* which was made into a highly successful movie. The

Rubin volume that naturally interested us the most was his *Thin Book by a Formerly Fat Psychiatrist* (Trident Press). It's perhaps the only nontechnical book around that manages to come to terms with the often overwhelming psychological problems involved in the arduous process of taking weight off and (what's really tough) *keeping* it off.

The book was clearly written from the heart. It contains such neat little gimmicks as lists of "Ammunition Foods" (almost no calories), "Comfort Foods" (up-filling and not too sinful) and "Poison Foods" (stay away!). But its unique contribution is in its discussion of food for the soul—specifically the dieter's notoriously weak willpower. (Sample: "It is the time and work and struggle involved in getting thin that will reestablish your image and your eating habits as well as your morale and your sense of self-reliance and responsibility for self.")

It sounded autobiographical, and it was.

Back during his Brooklyn childhood Ted Rubin had been a big, strong, outgoing kid with an absolutely wolfish appetite. He measured six feet three inches at the age of 14, easily wrestled as many as three other kids to the floor simultaneously and ate as many as ten small lamb chops at a single sitting. "I was working in my father's drugstore," he recalled, "and I think I ate with every customer who came in."

With a hyperactive life his weight nevertheless stayed for years at a nicely skinny 156 pounds. Then, during medical school in Lausanne, Switzerland, his weight gradually went up to 215 pounds. The life was sedentary, and Ted Rubin found that the less he slept, the more he ate. Food—and he quickly became a connoisseur of Swiss cuisine—was his reaction to fatigue. The trouble got worse during his internship when he ran a hectic emergency room at Santa Monica Hospital in Los Angeles and often didn't sleep for twenty-four or thirty-six hours.

"I ate to get boosts of energy," he said. "They served sandwiches all day long, so I ate all day long."

His eating pattern was set. "When I was interning, I used to eat three hamburgers and a double malted at one sitting," the doctor continued, smiling wistfully at the recollection. "I could go to an Italian restaurant for an Italian dinner and then have a Chinese meal right after that in a Chinese place. I remember in Chicago I once had a steak dinner in one place and then a complete spaghetti dinner in another place fifteen minutes later."

The doctor's wife, Eleanor, who also watches her weight, mentioned at this point that her husband has stayed very much interested not only in quantity of food over the years but in quality as well. "He's a gourmet eater," she said. "What he likes, he likes the best of. I mean, he has a lot of low-down tastes like hot dogs and pizza, but it always has to be the best." In short, Ted Rubin is the type of eater who even today will travel to an obscure restaurant in a way-out-of-the-way section of Brooklyn because he is convinced that the place serves the best steaks in Greater New York.

Settling down to his practice in psychiatry in Manhattan, Dr. Rubin repeatedly went on crash diets. At least three times he lost between twenty and thirty pounds. Gradually, he always regained all the lost weight. "In those days I did it mostly because of vanity," he said. "I looked like a fat man, and I didn't like it."

But the gorging instinct was stronger than mere vanity. Ted Rubin kept devouring enormous quantities of pastrami, sour cream, banana splits and other whipped cream desserts, malteds ("I was great on malteds—usually with pretzels. Pretzels—yup, pretzels!"). He ate two eggs for breakfast every morning, lots of beef at lunch and dinner and relatively little fish.

Then, twelve years ago, a number of things happened in the doctor's life that changed his food habits for good. First, he began to notice how many relatively young people of his acquaintance were dying of coronaries. Next, there was a certain evening when the Rubins had a visit from some neighbors. As Mrs. Rubin remembered: "We were looking through some old pictures in our family album, and there was Ted when he was a deck officer in the Navy, about the same time we got married. And the lady who was visiting us was saying, 'My God, Ted, you were so *handsome* when you were thin!' " The remark stung.

What really turned the tide, however, was the doctor's own physical state. He felt sluggish, tired. He was short of breath. He had terrific gas pains much of the time. Then, his internist diagnosed a condition that, in lay terms, is best described as "premature heart-beats." Dr. Rubin described its effects like this: "It's like the breath is knocked out of you; as if your heart stops. It's uncomfortable, and it makes you awfully conscious that you have a heart. As soon as I lost weight, it stopped."

The onset of his heart condition finally convinced the doctor that his next diet would have to have permanent results. "I finally made up my mind to do it," he said, "and I put Elly on notice that this time it was going to be a serious venture." That meant that this time there was careful preparation. For instance, Dr. Rubin made certain that he would not start dieting on a weekend, when he might have time on his hands ("That would be very hard"), but on a normal week-day when he would be very busy and wouldn't have time to think of his food self-deprivations.

By this time, too, the doctor's previous diets had taught him a great deal about his diet "hang-ups" (the expression is his, not ours) and what to do about them:

1. Knowing that much of his extra eating was a response to fatigue, he tried not to get too tired too often, thereby making himself less vulnerable.

2. He knew he had to have some kind of food available in quantity for the occasions when he simply *had* to "fill up," so he asked his wife to cook up "huge quantities" of fresh mushrooms and marinated onions and always to have on hand a plentiful supply of sour pickles, carrots, bean sprouts, celery and other very-low-calorie foods.

3. He watched himself with special care during times of unusual tension and anxieties.

4. He now realized that permanent weight loss would require an extended, slow "campaign," not the crash principle he had tried before.

5. "I knew I had to take vacations from dieting, so I contracted with myself that if I could just sustain my weight losses during my 'rest periods,' it would be a victory." Over a year, then, Dr. Rubin lost more than 50 pounds, 10 pounds at a time, with "vacations" after every 10 pounds. Since then he has weighed as little as 190 pounds, which is exemplary for a man of his height and his vast bone structure.

Today it's still a battle. When we interviewed the

doctor, he was forty-five, mustached, balding, quick-spoken, emphatic, and he smiled often. His weight was 204 pounds, but "I'd like to be one ninety-five." The most significant item about the doctor's weight over the past dozen years, however, is that he has never again climbed over 207 pounds. In order to maintain this record, he periodically restricts his now normal diet even further. He does this every three months, always for a period of two months at a time.

"Overweight is controllable but not curable," he said. "The trick is not to let it get malignant, but to get it while it's benign."

For breakfast these days Dr. Rubin normally has grapefruit juice, some tuna fish with lemon juice (either water-pack or with the oil carefully drained off), and tea and nothing else. Sometimes he has a three-ounce steak instead of the fish. Since he practices in the large, comfortable brownstone off Fifth Avenue where he also lives, he eats lunch at home. Often he has "a lot" of shrimp or scallops or a seafood salad and a "big" dessert of low-calorie gelatine or pudding. Between meals he usually has from six to eight cups of hot tea a day, a hangover from childhood customs. "If I'm desperate I'll have half a cantaloupe with pot cheese." At dinner there now is much veal, chicken, much less beef, and steak only once a week.

There are no desserts except fruit or dietetic gelatines and puddings in this house, and the doctor has virtually eliminated bread, along with most of his other favorites, like pastrami.

"On Sundays maybe I'll have half a bagel," he said.

"Pastrami?" said Mrs. Rubin. "I never bring it into the house."

The Rubins do not have much taste for alcoholic drinks. The doctor likes one twenty-five-year-old Ambassador Scotch on the rocks every other day or so and sometimes daily, but he has no trouble cutting even this ration during his periods of more restricted intake. Mrs. Rubin prefers Manhattans made with Jack Daniel bourbon, but she indulges only when she is entertaining or the Rubins are invited out.

The Rubins do have pre-bedtime snacks. When they are not restricting themselves particularly, the doctor may have cantaloupe and pot cheese, and his wife will nibble on an apple and some hard cheese. During their leaner periods it's animal crackers and tea for both the doctor and his wife, and that's all. "It's the highlight of our evening," said Eleanor Rubin ruefully.

For a long time now she has bought butter only when there was company; bacon and American cheese only for their six-year-old son (the Rubins also have a boy of twenty and a daughter of seventeen); no cookies except vanilla wafers and animal crackers; only skim or buttermilk; no ice cream or ice cream substitutes;

and very little more bread than is needed to keep the housekeeper happy.

At that, Mrs. Rubin still has a weight problem. At forty-two, she weighed 150 pounds (her height is five feet eight inches), but at age sixteen she had weighed 165 ("More than my brother-in-law! I was so shocked that I went straight down to 135"). When her husband made his big diet change twelve years ago, she weighed 142 pounds. Unfortunately, Mrs. Rubin confesses to a fatal weakness for chocolate marshmallow wafers and other kinds of chocolate candy. "Especially Hershey kisses," she said. "I'll buy a big bag, supposedly for the kids, and then on my way home from the super market I find myself . . ."

When we met Mrs. Rubin, she expected once again to slim down, hopefully with the help of the low-calorie gourmet recipes in her own new book, *The Doctor's Wife's Thinking Thin Cookbook* (Trident Press), which contains many of the dishes that make her husband's belt-tightening periods bearable.

Dr. Rubin feels guilty about not getting more exercise. "I'm no sports enthusiast," he said. "Golf looks moronic to me. I envy people who get involved in these things. More power to them!" The doctor walks as much as he feels he has time for—usually forty or fifty blocks a couple of times a week—but he confessed, "What I really like is to play poker."

He is satisfied with his settled-down dietary regimen, although he admits feeling somewhat martyred in the knowledge that he can have a luscious hot dog or a pastrami sandwich only once every three or four months. "It's part of the unfairness of life," he said with a grin. "I must say I envy those people who seem to stay thin with little trouble. They're really sporadic eaters. It's just that when you catch them it *looks* as if they can eat anything." He sighed.

9

DR. COHN : *Life Is Just a Bowl of Nibbles*

For some unknown reason Dr. Clarence Cohn has never felt like eating very much on any one occasion. "After an appetizer, soup and salad, I'm about ready to call it quits," he says. But for most of his adult life Dr. Cohn has also been an inveterate nibbler, ever eager to enjoy a small snack outside of traditional meal hours. This casual regimen obviously has been good for him. At fifty-five, this clinical pathologist is director of the Division of Nutritional Sciences at Michael Reese Hospital in Chicago. His weight ranges between 170 and 175 pounds, just a little above his World War II army weight of 168 (Dr. Cohn is six feet tall). And, somewhat to his embarrassment, his eating habits have become the subject of lively discussion among diet experts. Quite a few doctors are starting to believe that we should perhaps all eat like Dr. Cohn and that someday many of us will.

The serious medical interest in Dr. Cohn's nibbling developed not long after the doctor began to subject his habits to scientific scrutiny in 1962. Although his wife, Pauline, keeps joshing her husband about his professional interest in snacking ("Clarie invented a theory to fit his eating habits"), the doctor did not really consider himself a guinea pig. He is a distinguished-looking man, erect and courtly, with a distinct resemblance to Rudy Vallee. He is also a distinguished researcher, an exceptionally precise person who will tell you in exhaustive detail something he did "one and a quarter years" ago. Nobody would think of accusing him of frivolity or of trying to inject an undue personal element into his work.

The reasoning behind Dr. Cohn's first experiment is described by him, with typical self-deprecation, as "naïve." He simply noted that nobody had ever come up with a cogent medical reason why anybody should live on three meals a day. Most babies, in fact, eat only when they feel like it, and seem to satisfy their appetites and needs for oral gratification quite nicely that way. After conducting numerous experiments with chickens, rabbits and rats, Dr. Cohn decided to test the effects of snacking on a group of human volunteers.

He recruited six normal eaters ("free eaters") and matched them against six comparable subjects who were required to live on six relatively small meals a day. The total number of calories consumed by each group was the same. Dr. Cohn was not interested in weight loss as a specific goal. He was concerned principally with body fat and the general health and happiness of his subjects.

The results were arresting. Psychologists who had not been informed of the experiment's purpose and did not know that they were dealing with two groups, administered tests to the guinea pigs before the experiment began and after it ended. They found that the snackers had turned distinctly "happier" than the free eaters. Even more remarkable, four out of six snackers experienced a drop in their blood cholesterol levels, and several reported that while their weight remained unchanged their waistlines were reduced by from one to one and one-half inches. Their biggest complaint about the experiment was that their belts had become too loose!

As his research progressed, Dr. Cohn refined his

eating habits in line with the results of his experiments. He also encouraged his wife and his three daughters, aged twelve to sixteen, to become snackers. For example, Dr. Cohn had long ago reduced his egg consumption to one per week (always on Sunday morning). He had been breakfasting on fruit or juice, one slice of toast with margarine and orange marmalade, and black coffee. Now he *added* a dish of cold cereal (usually two or three different kinds that he mixed himself) and skim milk.

"Man usually eats most of his protein at night," he said. "We found that the rat grows less well that way, although it makes for a fatter rat. The more one spreads out the protein, the better it's utilized." For the same reason, the Cohn children may eat some leftover roast beef for breakfast, and their morning meal often resembles a very small dinner.

Like most of the doctors we interviewed, Dr. Cohn is a restless man, always mobile, always exuding energy. Like quite a few of his colleagues he seems, for instance, constitutionally unable to sit still for more than a few seconds at a time. He is forever shifting his head, his legs, his arms, his chair. His work schedule would break any man who is not in top condition. He is up six days a week at 5:15 A.M. Unless it rains, he walks one mile to the station from his suburban Winnetka home. At the hospital he has no mid-morning snack, and his lunch is hardly magnificent: usually soup, cottage cheese and a tomato with French dressing or else a hamburger or a frankfurter.

"If I'm bored, I will get hungry in the afternoon," he said, "but I'm never sitting behind the desk worrying, 'Now it's time to eat.' I run around a lot, and it keeps my mind off things."

At the same time Dr. Cohn also has to cope with an unconquerable sweet tooth. He is enormously fond of chocolate cake, which he now eats only on Sundays. For years, however, he has enjoyed a candy bar daily in the late afternoon, and this is a treat he refuses to give up. "He's a sweet eater," said his wife. "When he is trying to lose weight, he has eliminated entire meals, but not sweets."

At dinnertime the Cohns have cut down on fats. The doctor always cuts some meat off with the fat when he trims a steak on his plate. Butter, said Mrs. Cohn, "is mostly for the maid." There is none for dinner unless fresh corn is served, and there are only two slices of bread on the table. "One for me and one to go back to the kitchen," said Mrs. Cohn.

The hold-down on fats is not as rigorous here as it is in the homes of some other doctors. Home-fried potatoes are considered a relatively rare treat, but they have not become extinct. Bacon is served with liver. Lasagne and French fried shrimp are among the standard entrées. So are spaghetti with meat sauce, stuffed mushrooms and hot dogs. Even French fried potatoes appear once every three weeks or so. The Cohns do not happen to be concerned about liquor, and they have cocktails only when there are guests. Normal consumption is one small glass of wine for Friday night dinner. ("Alcohol is a lost cause in our house.")

The chief difference between dinner at the Cohns' and the same meal at the home of other diet experts is in the size of the portions: The Cohns have trained themselves to eat even less than the others. One fryer weighing two and a half pounds is enough for five; so are hamburgers made from a pound and a quarter of lean ground beef. Mrs. Cohn never gets standing rib roasts ("They're much too fat"). She uses sirloin tip, and four and a half pounds of it yield two full meals for the entire family, plus a few sandwiches.

How do the Cohns last through the evening? Simply by more snacking. Unlike most of the doctors we interviewed, the Cohns have not eliminated desserts. They serve dessert as a separate meal around 9 P.M., and pie as well as ice cream are standard dishes, along with fruit. The doctor and his wife help themselves to coffee throughout the evening, and between 10 and 11 P.M. Dr. Cohn always enjoys a melted Swiss-cheese sandwich—another deliberate step designed to spread out protein consumption as much as possible throughout the waking hours.

Mrs. Cohn has applied the snacking techniques to herself so that she estimates she consumes about two thousand calories a day—just right so that she will not gain weight. However, at the time of our interview she had not yet succeeded in snacking away any excess poundage. At forty-seven and five feet six inches tall, she weighs 142 pounds, compared with 116 pounds at the time of her marriage nineteen years ago. Mrs. Cohn, who holds a degree in medical technology and who met her husband not long after both started working at Michael Reese Hospital, attributes her weight problems to emotional causes triggered by serious illness and surgery.

Her attitude toward the very act of stepping on the scale is characteristic of someone with a continuing weight problem. While her husband weighs himself twice or more each week on a medical scale, Pauline Cohn cheerfully confessed: "If I eat a lot, I don't weigh myself. If I'm in the mood to lose weight, then I weigh myself once a day."

Her usual breakfast consists of fruit, coffee with skim milk and a piece of cheese—nothing else. At ten-thirty she has some bread with a cold cut or cheese. At noon another piece of bread with meat or cheese. At 2 P.M., if she is hungry, she will have half a piece of bread with meat or cheese and perhaps a tomato. At four-thirty she has a piece of fruit. Then comes dinner with the family, the separate "meal" of dessert with the family, and at bedtime another nibble of bread and meat.

The children have taken to their parents' eating patterns without much, if any, difficulty, quite possibly because their new way of handling food allows them to eat pretty much all the time. Dr. Cohn has taken further steps to reduce their fat intake ("I don't like them smearing oleo or butter all over their bread, and we no longer give them milk before they go to sleep"), but the art of keeping their snacks small has largely been absorbed by the children as a matter of habit and, as their mother said, "because they see their parents eat that way."

Astoundingly, when one of the children helps herself to an éclair at dessert time, she may well eat only half and say, "I'll have the rest later." Mrs. Cohn reported: "Like ourselves, these kids cannot eat a big meal. We have candy around the house, but it's not consumed. And if they make themselves an ice-cream cone, they'll take small scoops because I never gave them big ones."

10

DR. PAGE : *An Elder Statesman's Diet*

Dr. Irvine H. Page was chatting with a group of fellow guests at a cocktail party some years ago when another guest stepped up and quickly overheard that the subject under discussion happened to be seaweeds.

"Oh?" said the newcomer. "How do you cook them?"

Dr. Page hastily explained that he had never tasted seaweeds in any form and had only been pointing out what they were doing to the coast of Cape Cod, where he owns a summer house.

As misunderstandings go, this one was instructive.

It illustrates that diet-conscious citizens will grasp at almost any straw (or weed) if they think it could somehow help them take off weight, and that any word from Dr. Page about food inspires automatic interest and confidence.

Such faith is entirely understandable in view of Dr. Page's stature in his profession. He is a former president of the American Heart Association and director of the government's National Diet-Heart Study. His own research into the relationship between diet and heart disease has made him famous throughout the world and landed him, among many other honorable places, on the cover of *Time* magazine. As director of research for the highly regarded Cleveland Clinic until his recent retirement, he occupied one of the most prestigious spots in American medicine. He now serves as senior consultant to the clinic.

Appropriately, Dr. Page is something of a patrician figure. At sixty-six, he weighed in at an enviable 146 pounds (his height is five feet ten). His ample gray hair is brushed straight back. His posture is exemplary. His movements are smooth and economical; it is obvious that he is not the type of man who wastes a second if he can help it. A movie producer might consider casting him as a general staff officer planning a major invasion, but he would probably change his mind once he heard Dr. Page talk at some length about his own diet problems. Perhaps he is a little too human, after all. True, the doctor is hardly the emotional type, and his food tastes are quite uncomplicated ("I'm the despair of gourmets"). But he has learned by tedious personal experience that model eating habits are not easy to establish. He has become genuinely sympathetic toward eaters who find dietary sacrifices deeply painful. And he manages to sound considerably more relaxed about the whole subject than he did in the past.

None of this is unrelated to the circumstance that Dr. Page had a diet problem himself. At the time of World War II he weighed almost twenty pounds more than he does now: 164, to be exact, and he remembers the figure well. And while his blood cholesterol level now stands at 222, it had risen as high as 310 in the early 1950's, which is a decidedly elevated reading.

A few years previously Dr. Page had become professionally interested in the role of cholesterol in heart disease, and his early scientific findings caused him to take some heroic measures to mend his own ways. He completely cut out all table spreads, eggs, cheese, ice cream, whole milk, pork, bacon and other fatty meats. He gave up all baked goods ("I used to like sweet rolls and cookies"). He even made what was for him the supreme sacrifice: He renounced peanut butter.

"I used to be very fond of peanut butter," the doctor said, still a bit wistful after all these years. "Every night before going to bed I had a big peanut-butter sandwich. I gave it up with great reluctance." He also very much liked all sorts of egg and cheese dishes, especially cheese soufflés, and concedes that he found it "a little frustrating" to give up all such goodies.

At one point during the period of his early research (and his most rigorous dieting), Dr. Page was almost never eating anything for lunch except a dish of cottage cheese with catsup. By that time only 15 percent of his calories were derived from fats, and the doctor frequently felt bloated because of carbohydrate fermentation.

"I wasn't having any fun, that's for sure," he recalled. "People used to kid hell out of me. They thought I was nuts. And they could have been right."

As the years went by and further research results began to accumulate, from work at the Cleveland Clinic as well as at many other centers, Dr. Page relaxed his regimen considerably.

"If all Americans had a cholesterol of a hundred fifty, it would be very nice," he said, "but I don't think it's all that important. I've become much less compulsive about it."

Today Dr. Page does eat sherbet and cookies and "an occasional slice" of bread with jam or jelly. He drinks more than a quart of skim milk a day ("I really *like* milk"). He uses cream in his coffee again ("a trace: just enough to color it") and any kind of salad dressing that "comes along." He eats a little more beef, perhaps, and has not increased his fish consumption (he likes fish, but his family doesn't). Still, to follow him through a day of typical menus is not a form of exercise that we would recommend to, say, a French chef.

Dr. Page habitually breakfasts at 5 A.M. The menu: shredded wheat in a bowl full of corn flakes (with skim milk) and a cup of coffee. "This is the breakfast I enjoy," he said. He lunches at eleven-thirty, usually at the clinic and usually on nothing more than a fruit salad and a package of crackers. Before dinner the doctor enjoys a stiff (two-ounce) drink of bourbon or Scotch on the rocks. Dinner itself is a normal meal except for what most Americans would consider downright parsimonious portions. At bedtime Dr. Page has a snack of cold cereal and skim milk, and sometimes there is a similar snack between dinner and bedtime.

His dignity notwithstanding, the doctor is a gregarious person who enjoys putting other people at their ease and, unlike some of our more stern-minded interviewees, does not like his food habits to interfere with sociability. At a dinner party he refuses no food, although he does report: "You don't eat so much at a party. They always take my plate away when I'm busy talking." To preserve the amenities at home, his wife, Beatrice, cooks for guests just as any other well-to-do hostess would. Shrimp creole is one of Mrs. Page's specialties. Another is beef stroganoff in sour cream. She also serves buttered rolls at parties and such desserts as chocolate cake and éclairs.

"Sometimes I eat seconds just to make the guests feel comfortable," she said.

Smoking continues to be a far more serious problem, both for the doctor and for Mrs. Page. Dr. Page smoked a pack of cigarettes a day until about ten years ago. Then he cut down to fifteen per day. Then he switched to filter cigarettes. Then to filter holders. About four years ago he stopped all smoking until the cocktail hour, and he then limits himself to four cigarettes for the rest of the day ("unless I happen to be out at some big shindig"). As he analyzed it, "I'm sure I smoke for companionship. It wouldn't occur to me to smoke when I'm alone."

Mrs. Page, who has published one novel and is working on another, was smoking a pack and a half a day in 1950 and now is down to about 15 cigarettes a day, "sometimes less but never more than a pack," and she rarely smokes until after lunch.

"I don't suffer to keep my weight down, like many people I know," said the tall, elegant Mrs. Page, who weighs 125 pounds and never weighed more than 128 in her life. "I can feel every pound over a hundred twenty-two, and I just don't like the feeling. But I have great sympathy for others. I find it difficult to keep my smoking down, and it must be the same for people who like to eat. It's easy for us who don't have this weakness to talk about self-discipline."

But self-discipline, as Dr. Page sees it, is by no means the entire answer to the problem of eating less; wifely cooperation is another key, and the doctor, like just about every one of our experts, picked himself a good working partner thirty-six years ago. "I don't miss any foods anymore," he said. "As long as you've got somebody who cooperates, these things work themselves out. Neither one of us feels put upon."

In the Page family the doctor does nearly all the marketing. "He just enjoys it," said his wife, who disclaims any great interest in culinary affairs and often feels slightly guilty about her indifference. ("Even making a sandwich is such a bore for me.") The doctor does not mind buying such items as eggs (his wife has one, poached on toast, every morning) and even Muenster cheese, also mostly for his wife. But the quantities that he purchases, especially at the meat counter, would startle most homemakers.

A few days before our interview, Mrs. Page recalled, her sons, Christopher, twenty-five, and Nicholas, twenty-three, were not at home, and she and her husband shared a sirloin tip roast. "We had three pounds, which lasted three nights, with leftovers for lunches," she said. "A leg of lamb lasts forever in this family. Say it's six pounds. We have it roasted the first night, sliced cold the next night, then we have a stew or curry that takes us two nights to eat up. Also, usually one of the boys gets a sandwich. And the cat is very fond of lamb. We also make a meat loaf for four from one pound of lean ground chuck, with some left over."

Considering his age, Dr. Page's devotion to regular exercise is a pointed reminder to the rest of us that he and his colleagues really consider physical exertion important to good health. Like everybody else, the doctor is not enamored of calisthenics and does only about two or three minutes' worth a day (knee bends, arm swings, leg lifts), always before he takes his predinner shower, but he has been holding these blitz sessions for more than a decade, and he does so every day. For forty years Dr. Page has also been playing tennis, usually indoors and on Saturdays as well as Sundays. Normally he plays at least three sets, often four. Finally, like so many of our experts, the doctor looks upon walking with the kind of enthusiasm that the rest of us reserve for a favorite TV series or a particularly cherished dessert.

"I enjoy walking," he said. "The clinic is a seven-story building, and I never take an elevator. I also don't like to take cabs if I can avoid it, and I try to avoid picking up the telephone as often as I can. I much prefer to talk to a person face to face."

Mrs. Page, a former professional dancer who studied modern dance in Germany, encountered an unexpected opportunity to give her own exercise program a renewed push five years ago. "I can't *bear* ordinary calisthenics," she said, although she had long been trying valiantly to stick with a daily sequence of warm-up exercises, which she does with the help of recorded music. Then a group of friends and acquaintances, who also felt they should be getting more exercise, asked her to start classes in basic ballet and modern dance. She did and now teaches a group of eighteen women.

"I had no intention of teaching," Mrs. Page said. "I was pushed into it. Now I'm terribly glad, and I feel much better for it."

Being careful about food is not difficult for Mrs. Page. She is usually up before 5 A.M. and starts working on her writing while still in bed. A pint of coffee is always nearby, and she may nibble on some Metrecal cookies. The coffee is flavored with Sucaryl and milk made from nonfat milk solids. Her breakfast egg is not only never fried or scrambled, but about six years ago Mrs. Page began to leave most of the yolk on her plate to avoid cholesterol. Lunch may be fresh fruit and cottage cheese, or a slice of cheese on white bread, popped into the oven. "If there are leftovers, I feel duty-bound to get them out of the way," she said, "and sometimes I'll have frozen strawberries on some cottage cheese. That sort of gives you the feeling you're eating dessert, too." During the afternoon and often at other times Mrs. Page nibbles on cookies with coffee or skim milk. Before dinner she joins her husband for two drinks of bourbon on the rocks (Tom Collins or gin and tonic in summer).

Her dinner menus are simple but not monotonous. Standard lean meats and poultry are the mainstays, but "I'm always on the lookout for simple casseroles." Chicken with artichoke hearts, meatballs and noodles, and veal in creole sauce are among her favorites.

Neither of the Page sons has a weight problem. "When they were little, they ate a lot," Mrs. Page recalled. "I tried to limit them, and I was the ogre many times, but I suppose they ate as much as other kids." Neither boy was particularly fond of athletics, but both love to dance and play tennis, and they did not mind mowing their parents' sizable lawn with a hand mower.

"I think children will pick these things up," said Dr. Page. "I don't think we really began thinking about these children's diets until they were twelve or thirteen. Nick went through a peanut-butter stage when he was about seven or eight, but he finally grew out of it." As we observed in other doctors' families, children are lucky when they grow up in a household where "eating lean" is the more or less natural thing because of parental habits. The youngsters do indeed tend to "pick these things up." Dr. Page has one fascinating memory that makes this process of natural absorption particularly clear.

When the family cat, Skipper, who was fifteen at the time of our interview, was only two months old, the doctor switched her dietary mainstay from whole milk to skim milk and also began to feed her other low-fat foods. His sons asked him about it, and he explained briefly that he was making the change to prolong the cat's life.

"Kids remember that," the doctor said.

P.S. In June 1967, Dr. Page suffered a heart attack. When colleagues and reporters asked him for a self-diagnosis of its cause, he attributed it to life-long immoderation in his work habits. He did not indict overwork or tension but excessive drive. "I was continually dissatisfied," he said. "I always tried to drive myself harder." This he now recognized was a mistake. His diet and exercise patterns were not. "Who knows?" he said. "Without good health practices I might have had an attack earlier, or my attack might have been more severe." At this writing, Dr. Page was considerably more relaxed—and feeling fine.

11

DR. ANCEL KEYS : *Eating Lean, the High-Style Way*

In all probability Dr. Ancel Keys of Minneapolis is the best-known of the experts we interviewed, and we had heard quite a lot about him. He was one of the earliest and most vociferous critics of the average American's consumption of fats. Years before most of us first encountered the very word "cholesterol," Dr. Keys was speaking up among his fellow experts on the dangers of living with too much of this fatty substance in the blood. He kept pointing out large population groups in various parts of the world who ate a diet low in animal fats and turned out to have low blood cholesterol levels—and, evidently by no coincidence, far less heart and artery disease than those of us living on typical American diets.

Dr. Keys, we knew, had an impeccable record as a researcher. He had taught at Cambridge and Oxford Universities, had been an adviser to the World Health Organization, and held such offices as the vice chairmanship of the International Society of Cardiology. His face had even been on the cover of *Time* Magazine. But he was also controversial, often attacked for his caustic manner and widely admired for the courage that his critics dismissed as gall.

Certainly it had not been easy for the doctor to lead, in effect, a national crusade against butter and other dairy products from his headquarters as director of the Laboratory of Physiological Hygiene at the University of Minnesota's School of Public Health, smack in the middle of a state whose economy is heavily dependent on the prosperity of its dairy farms. We had heard complaints from other diet researchers that Dr. Keys was a notoriously difficult man to argue with, principally because of the ambitious size of population studies that he had been running for many years in such countries as Japan, Italy and Finland. His statistical evidence was just too convincing for comfort.

"Ancel can talk back with his case material every time," one of the doctor's Eastern admirers had told us.

It is no exaggeration to say that much diet research in the past decade has been undertaken throughout the United States as specific efforts to prove Dr. Keys wrong.

We knew that Dr. Keys is an impressive fellow on other counts as well. He is a mushroom collector and a recognized authority on port wine. With his wife, Margaret, a biochemist, he wrote one the best of the modern diet books, *Eat Well and Stay Well* (Doubleday), which contains some ingenious low-fat gourmet recipes we had used ourselves. Finally, we had been made aware that Dr. Keys loves to eat and talk about fine food.

Other doctors had told us, "Wait till you have one of Ancel's candlelight dinners." The male member of this reporting team was therefore delighted to be asked for an evening meal at the doctor's large, beautiful, lakeshore home, which is surrounded by professional-looking stone walls that were erected by the doctor personally.

Like most reformers basking in the ever-increasing acceptance of their peers, Dr. Keys turned out to be agreeable, untroubled by his critics and clearly enjoying himself. At sixty-three, he is in splendid shape (height: five feet six and a half inches, weight 160). His weight has never been higher than 168. His blood cholesterol level has been as high as 208, which is exemplary, and now registers at a stunningly low 186. He weighs himself once a week and has his cholesterol checked once a year.

However, like so many of his colleagues, he is hardly a relaxed man. His aristocratic face, the elegant manner and the authoritative voice don't impress you as much as the doctor's physical voltage. When Ancel Keys gets you a Scotch and soda, he does not walk into the kitchen. He storms in and out of his library, so that you can almost see the stirring of the air around his coattails.

Dinner under the Keys candles lasted about two hours and was a delight. Beforehand, Mrs. Keys, who is clearly accustomed to letting her articulate husband bring off a dazzling solo performance, had served what tasted like—but wasn't—an excellent Roquefort-cheese dip. In point of fact, it was concocted of dry curd cottage cheese, mixed in the blender with nonfat milk, onion juice, minced clams, a dash of salt and one small chunk of blue cheese. In the dining room there was good conversation, much of it about various other diet experts, and not all of it complimentary; beef broth pastini, boiled beef that looked so lean that all its fat seemed to have been blown clean away by some new and mysterious process, peppers with eggplant and tomatoes, and a flawless bottle of wine.

Wine is important to Dr. Keys. He has given up all other liquor for caloric reasons, and he does not drink at lunch except for a small glass of wine when he is in Italy, where he is building a home for his retirement. But good wine at dinner is just about indispensable to his welfare. ("When I'm faced with dinner without wine, it's like some sort of punishment. We usually kill a bottle between the two of us.")

Perhaps the tastiest and most resourceful touch with the dinner was the sauce for the beef. Almost none of the wives of our other experts ever bother with sauce. Indeed, many take pride in having banished sauce permanently from their households. Dr. and Mrs. Keys, to whom austerity is an unacceptable insult, manage to reconcile their high-taste preferences with the low-fat requirement that they feel is the key to healthy eating. Mrs. Keys had made a sauce of chopped parsley mixed with corn oil, vinegar and lemon juice. It was superb, and Dr. Keys's comment would have gladdened the heart of any glutton.

"It's best when you take a lot," he said.

None of this was a special show for the benefit of a guest. Dr. and Mrs. Keys are concerned about the aesthetics of food. They care about making it special. Unlike most of the other experts, they have elevated food to play an important role in their lives, and do not mind admitting it.

"We talk all the time about food," the doctor said. "We can have dinner by ourselves for two and a half hours and are capable of spending half that time talking about food. Perhaps it is partly sublimation for actual eating. And we do eat very slowly. The majority of people I know who are seriously obese are fast eaters."

Oddly enough, Dr. Keys's sophisticated palate made it easier for him to switch his diet into a low-fat pattern, beginning more than ten years ago. He grew up in San Francisco and learned to like Chinese and Italian cooking, which is generally sparing in the use of animal fats. After he was married, there was never much butter around the house, and there were never any creamy cakes and pies. In the early 1950's there still used to be some butter on the table, but even then the older of the two Keys daughters, now married, used to ask for it by saying, "Please pass the poison." Not long after that, butter disappeared in the Keys home.

"There is only one occasion a year when I buy butter," said Mrs. Keys. "That's for my Béarnaise sauce for the salmon on New Year's Eve. I just can't do it without butter."

Luckily, Dr. Keys had no major problem with eggs. He never had them for breakfast except occasionally on Sundays, and even then he preferred such treats as popovers and waffles. Also, Mrs. Keys never did buy commercially baked products. She likes to bake strawberry-and-rhubarb pies, and estimates that she makes perhaps ten of them per year. Since about a decade ago she has been baking with vegetable oil. At about the same time she also started substituting cottage cheese for such cheeses as Mozzarella in cooking. The doctor still is fond of Provolone and used to serve it with cocktails, but he gave up this fatty extravagance. He also likes milk, and drinks about a pint a day, but he switched from regular to skim milk about seven years ago.

Dr. and Mrs. Keys eat less beef now than they used to (and never such fatty cuts as standing rib roasts). They still have pork tenderloin about twice a month. Chicken (usually roasted), veal roasts, beef tongue and beef hearts are more frequently on the menu than they used to be, and fish is now served once or twice a week, even though the doctor is not overly fond of it. Sherbet is served about twice a year, ice cream never, although the children were always allowed to eat it in school.

Over the years Dr. Keys also found that he had to give up some of his habits purely for caloric reasons in order to maintain his gourmet dinner tastes and still not gain weight. He used to have a bit of cake or bread or cookies with his "tea breaks" in the office.

Now he just has two cups of tea. About seven years ago he also gave up bedtime snacks. He now keeps two little plastic boxes on his bedside table. One contains almonds, and he may have four or five of them at bedtime. The other box holds dried apricots, and he usually nibbles on two or three. For practical purposes though, the doctor has cut out all between-meal eating.

He insists that none of this belt-tightening has caused him any pain, even though some of it occurred during the period when he stopped smoking. He used to smoke a pack of cigarettes a day and gave them up later than most of those medical men who have been able to wean themselves away from the habit. Dr. Keys stopped only about three years ago. Almost immediately he found himself going to lunch earlier than ever, even at such an ungourmetlike hour as 11:30 A.M. He also gained about five pounds and required more than a year to shed them.

Mrs. Keys, who smoked more than a pack a day, was having the same problems for the same reason and at approximately the same time. At fifty-six, she is five feet six and a half inches tall and weighs 140 pounds. Five years previously she weighed 130; ten years previously 125. At the time of our interview Mrs. Keys had not smoked for almost two years. She had just lost two pounds, and it had not been easy for her. To reverse her weight gains, she gave up all sec-

ond helpings and eliminated the cookies from her own
"tea break." About six years ago she also began a
personal program of daily exercise in addition to her
gardening (she does the lawn mowing and deliber-
ately uses a hand mower instead of a power mower)
and her traditional chores of taking care of her three-
story home.

The added daily exercise may not, offhand, sound
like much: a walk of from half an hour to three quar-
ters of an hour at a reasonably stiff pace, in the company of at least two neighbors and sometimes as many
as six. Mrs. Keys and her fellow walkers appreciate,
however, that exercise must be regular to be medically
useful, and so they really do walk every single week-
day unless the temperature sinks to ten degrees below
zero, which does not happen on too many days, even
in frigid Minnesota.

Dr. Keys, on the other hand, finds exercise a just
about insoluble problem these days. For years, while
he was building rock walls and mixing cement around
his home, his output of physical energy was so pro-
digious that he estimates he was keeping his trim figure
on four thousand calories a day. All in all, he believes
he handled about one hundred tons of stone as time
went by. He also used to do considerable long-distance
swimming. But now the construction projects are com-
pleted. Somehow he no longer finds the time for much

sport, and repetitive exercise just bores him too much ("The idea of doing jerk-ups would drive me nuts"). All of which is another major reason why he has had to restrict his eating.

The Keys family is another one where the children, growing up in a weight-conscious household, seemed to have far less difficulty with their figures than their parents ever did. None of the Keys children (aged twenty-six, twenty-three and seventeen) were ever made particularly conscious of any dietary restrictions, and they seem to have no weight problems. "Too active, I guess," their father said. Did he try to set a good example? "I have no idea," he snapped. "They swim and skate and chase around. I think most kids will eat okay if the food isn't pushed at them."

12

DR. FRANTZ : *A Physician in Search of a Cure*

Dr. Ivan S. Frantz is another of that relatively rare specimen: a diet expert with a chronic and serious weight problem. Actually, Dr. Frantz is expert at a good deal more than diets. He is George S. Clark Professor in the Departments of Medicine and Biochemistry at the University of Minnesota School of Medicine. He directs the school's justly famous cardiovascular laboratory. He is also one of the principal investigators, along with such other authorities as Drs. Keys and Stare, in the nationwide Diet-Heart Study, an ambitious government-financed program designed to furnish the final evidence to answer a still controversial question: Can heart disease be reduced in the population-at-large by feeding people a diet low enough in animal fats to make a difference, yet not so low as to make the diet unpalatable for the long pull?

As a top-ranking heart specialist, earnestly involved in this enormously expensive test, which may yet influence American eating habits for decades to come, Dr. Frantz felt he faced a personal dilemma. He takes great pride in his scientific objectivity and worries that his impartiality as a researcher might be endangered if he made major changes in his own diet on the basis of the present findings linking high-fat diets to heart disease.

"I just don't feel I can afford to defend radical changes before all the facts are in," he said, "and that may be ten or fifteen years more. In my own case, vanity has as much to do with my diet as health."

With these professional and philosophical considerations in the background, Dr. Frantz finds himself in the same situation as most Americans who are reluctant to make changes in their long-accustomed food habits and yet have reason to do something about their weight.

At the time of our interview Dr. Frantz, a quiet, soft-spoken man of fifty who measures five feet nine inches, weighed in at a trim 145 pounds. Three years before, however, he had weighed 165, his top weight, and in the previous twenty years had gone through two other cycles of gaining and then losing more than fifteen pounds. His blood cholesterol level stood at a low 200, and it had "never been high that I know of." But both of his parents had been overweight, which is often typical of people with especially stubborn weight problems.

The changes that Dr. Frantz made in his diet are particularly interesting in view of his insistence that the indictment against animal fats is still not solid and that his own diet adjustments were made purely for caloric reasons.

Dr. Frantz used to eat butter regularly, but he eats none now.

He used to drink two or three glasses of milk a day until about four years ago. Then he switched to skim milk. Then he cut out all milk.

He used to eat ice cream as often as once a day ("I *love* ice cream"), but now he takes only ice milk.

He has cut down drastically on his cheese intake and increased his fish consumption ("When I go out to dinner, which is very often for professional reasons, I almost always have fish").

He eats very few eggs because four years ago he cut out all breakfast except for a glass of orange juice.

His wife no longer buys prime meats; she uses only "choice."

Bacon, which is a favorite item for every member of his family, is now served only once every three weeks. Doughnuts, another favorite, appear only on Sundays, pound cake only once every two or three months.

The point is, of course, that for most Americans eating a typical diet, the easiest way to cut down on calories is to cut down on *all* fats and simply to ignore the controversy as to whether animal fats are particularly worrisome.

Incidentally, Dr. Frantz also is one of those doctors who believe that high salt intake may encourage high blood pressure. He therefore rarely puts extra salt on his food. "After a few weeks I didn't notice the difference," he said.

Dr. Frantz normally lunches at a business meeting. He usually has a hamburger or a hot dog or a fish sandwich and a cola drink, but about twice a week he is likely to have a full meat-and-potatoes meal. He often has dessert, normally melon or other fruit, but he takes no coffee breaks and no snacks during the day. ("In the office I'm just so busy I don't have time to think about eating.") He never drinks alcoholic beverages except on social occasions. His dinner is a conventional meal, although there usually is no bread and butter on the table, and two pounds of ground round or chuck will feed his entire family, including his five sons, aged eight to twenty-one.

When Dr. Frantz was taking off his excess poundage at the rate of two pounds a week, he was eating about twelve hundred calories a day, and his wife, Veronica ("Vee") used to cook specially for him, particularly such fresh vegetables as cabbage, cauliflower and broccoli, which the doctor was substituting for some of his normal meat intake. Now that he estimates he is eating two thousand to twenty-two hundred calories a day, no special cooking is necessary.

Dr. Frantz's most uncomfortable food problem comes after dinner. Like many of us, he is a night eater. Much of his work involves intensive study and writing, and he finds he performs best at these tasks between 10 P.M. and 1 A.M. He gets along on an average of about five hours of sleep, but he does not like to manage without snacking while he works at home, especially cookies and peanuts. "I'm liable to eat all through the evening," he confessed with a guilty smile, "That's my worst sin."

Exercise is another problem that he feels he has never mastered. His daytime work, like that of almost all doctors, involves considerable fast movement around hospital corridors, but Dr. Frantz is all too well aware that he should work out a good deal more than that. For a while he played tennis, but no more. "I don't like it," he said. "It's just a matter of wanting to do something else worse. I keep resolving that I'm going to take up golf, but I don't do it." It's not that he lacks interests outside of his work. He likes to spend time with his sons and is an expert ham radio operator (the antenna atop his house is twenty-five feet high). It's just, as he says regretfully, "I'm not a very active person. And then my wife is a very good cook."

Mrs. Frantz, who weighs only 105 pounds, does not share her husband's problem. "I've decided I'm just not going to get fat," she said. "Occasionally my weight does go up two or three pounds. But when I go up two pounds, I feel thick and awful."

Mrs. Frantz reflected, "Sometimes I think I eat all the time." She does. She has only coffee for breakfast; toast and coffee in midmorning; juice, cottage cheese and maybe soup for lunch; coffee or tea in the afternoon; hot milk and crackers at night. But, as is evident, she is another of our natural-born snackers; her "all-day eating" adds up to very few calories. And for dinner, a five-pound rolled roast lasts two evenings in the Frantz home, so it is obvious that all members of the family get along on modest portions.

Dr. and Mrs. Frantz reported that they faced no diet problems with any of their children. "I tend to be rather relaxed, to my wife's dismay," the doctor said.

"I don't even make the kids eat salad. I used to hate it. Now I love it and I think eventually they will, too. I don't even try to make them finish their vegetables. In a normal American household it's almost impossible to have nutritional deficiencies."

13

DR. BROWN : *When You Really Love Good Food*

"It drives you nuts," said Dr. Helen Brown. "It's usually something baked, and it's so good!"

Dr. Brown, the sixty-four-year-old director of dietary research at the Cleveland Clinic, was talking about one of her principal professional activities: food testing. Necessarily, hers is a life of unceasing temptation, and she is frank to confess that it is not solely a matter of doing a superior job at the clinic, where she has worked for 18 years. She is simply very fond of cooking well and eating well.

"I fuss around the kitchen gourmet style," she said. "It's fun to pick recipes from *The New York Times* and fix chicken tarragon and sautéed rice. It makes life a little more interesting."

It also imposes a severe strain on eating habits. Dr. Brown, a biochemist, is a brisk, bespectacled, somewhat professorial person with a deep and positive-sounding voice. She is hardly one of our leanest interviewees. She measures five feet six inches and weighs 158 pounds. This is a much improved showing over her weight in the early 1950's, when it climbed briefly ("and to my horror") to 170. Yet she is all too aware that it would be better for her to weigh less.

"Everyone has a weight problem, especially as they get older," she said. "Metabolically, your requirements decrease, but your appetite usually doesn't."

While Dr. Brown does not literally count calories, her training enables her to keep rather close track of the caloric values of everything she eats, which doesn't really make things easier. Over the past five years she reduced her intake from about two thousand calories daily to fourteen hundred or fifteen hundred but, unfortunately, this usually applies to weekdays only.

"Then I'm not near the refrigerator, so it's easy to go without," she said. "I fall down on weekends." This is the time when her gourmet instincts come to the fore. It is also the time when she eats desserts. And, especially, it's a time of eating more. "It's the quantity that matters more than anything else," she said.

Except for the nibbling that Dr. Brown must do in line of research duty, her daily food habits are conservative, and she has made determined efforts to cut down on animal fats and cholesterol. Her breakfast consists of an orange or juice, two slices of toast with a margarine that is particularly low in saturated fats, marmalade and black coffee. ("We used to get eggs by the dozen. Now we just have them occasionally for Sunday.") Her lunch is a sandwich (she eats only the meat or poultry, not the bread) or a salad and skim milk. Dinner, more often than not, is beef. ("I don't like to cook fish because of the odor.") However, instead of sirloin, Dr. Brown has switched to buying round steak, which she then tenderizes.

"I get the 'choice' grade, but only if they're lean," she said. "If they're fatty, I don't get them." She cooks only with oil, margarine and skim-milk solids. "I don't try consciously to skimp on the oil," she said, "but throwing in all that butter or cream is out."

Her only regular liquor consumption is a highball of Canadian Club and soda as a relaxing bedtime snack, usually with a few crackers.

The great bane of Dr. Brown's dietary life is her husband John, a lawyer who is five feet seven inches tall and weighed 160 pounds at the end of World War

II. Now, at sixty-two, he weighs only 145. "I look at him with great envy," said his wife. "He is able to push away from the dinner table. His portions are quite impressive to me. He just says, 'I'm eating too much,' and that's it. He never cheats, and he never takes seconds."

Mr. Brown has toast, juice and cereal for breakfast; a "businessman's lunch" such as knockwurst or liver and onions, usually with a bottle of beer; and dinner and late-night snacks along with his wife. However, he does eat *less* than she does (for example: only one slice of toast each morning), and this, plus perhaps a somewhat more efficient metabolism, makes the difference between his leanness and his wife's continual struggle.

The Browns make no special effort to get exercise ("We're *very* bad on that," said Dr. Brown. "It's so damned uninteresting"). Nevertheless, their two married daughters presumably picked up enough sound notions about good nutrition not to have developed any weight problems themselves.

"My daughter Peggy says her three-and-a-half-year-old is always asking for cookies," Dr. Brown reports. "So she gives him crackers. To him, they're cookies." It is the sort of small trick for which the doctor's grandson may someday turn out to be grateful.

"We always had treats around the house when the

children were growing up," said Mr. Brown. "But we had a little horror of root beer and that sort of stuff." He looked at his wife fondly and sympathetically. She smiled and sighed just a little.

14

DR. HELLERSTEIN : *Impatient Apostle of Exercise*

Dr. Herman Hellerstein is that rare, refreshing personality: the brilliant enthusiast, the nonconformist who knows how to articulate the case for a cause, the partisan who is sure that good sense is on his side, the lobbyist who is convinced that it's the rest of us who are out of step, not he—but that our unfortunate condition is simply not meant to last and won't. He *knows* that we'll all come around to his way of thinking. We just can't be foolish enough not to. He is the super-champion of exercise, and we defy anyone to talk to the doctor and come away without stepping a little faster, breathing a bit more deeply, and looking at man's surroundings with a fresh curiosity. Could it be that our environment is lying idly about us, a vast un-appreciated playground, waiting to be used to make us healthier, to help us feel more alive?

Dr. Hellerstein thinks so, and he is terribly con-vincing, probably because he arrived at his creed gradually and through years of his own research. He found his studies so persuasive that he seized on the results for himself and his family—and never had cause to regret it.

The doctor is a cardiologist and a professor of medi-cine at Western Reserve University in Cleveland and the University Hospitals there. He has been studying the role of exercise in the prevention of heart disease for more than fifteen years, and his work is among the most respected in this field. He talks scornfully of his arch enemies, what he indicts as the "gluttony" and "indolence" in the American way of life. He is fifty and looks very much younger. He measures five feet ten and three-quarter inches and has weighed no less than 163 and no more than 164 pounds for more than five years and never weighed more than 170. More-over, he finds it a little difficult to understand why any informed person should not live up to his standards.

His face is peaked, intense, mobile. His hair is

black and wavy. His body is forever on the move, even when he is sitting down. He is a thoroughly impatient man—the sort who will not tolerate television around his home because it would encourage inactivity among his six children—and it is not easy to summon up arguments against his logic.

"I believe in pleasurable things," he said. "I just don't think they should kill you."

Dr. Hellerstein started to change his eating habits earlier than most doctors and for a very personal reason. In the early 1940's, when he was an intern in Philadelphia, he found the hospital food so dreadful (and his income so close to nonexistent) that he subsisted mostly on eggs, omelets and cheese. He particularly loved Camembert, cream cheese and Provolone. "I was quite an expert on cheese at one time," he said. But then he read the very early research on cholesterol and began to wean himself away from these very high-fat foods. His resolution received a boost as early as 1946, when he was an assistant resident in pathology and (just like Dr. Bruce Taylor, the senior pathologist among our interviewees) became considerably disturbed by the fat that he discovered at autopsy in the arteries of patients who had died of heart disease.

By the time he was married the following year (his wife, Mary, is a pediatrician), there was no butter in his home (today the entire family uses less than a pound of margarine a week). Also, about 1947, the doctor stopped eating ice cream except as a treat, perhaps once every two and a half or three weeks, just as he did when his father took him to the drugstore back home in Dillonvale, Ohio, occasionally on Saturdays for a cone. ("There nothing wrong with ice cream. It's a matter of how often you use it.")

By 1950 the doctor began to make a conscious effort to substitute fish for meat at least once or twice a week and also started eating poultry two or three times a week. That year two other decisions were notable in his personal regimen: He was down to one visible egg a year (that is, an egg not used in cooking), and he had developed the habit of consuming this one egg at the annual meeting of the American Society of Arteriosclerosis just as a private joke. It was also that year when he began to appreciate the role of exercise in preventing heart attacks. He was asked to establish a clinic for the Cleveland Heart Society and, after studying several hundred cardiac patients, was struck by the way overweight, elevated blood pressure, elevated blood cholesterol levels and what he calls "indolence" seemed to march hand in hand.

By 1956 Dr. Hellerstein had begun to step up his efforts to get exercise, and he was doing so on a major scale. By now the campaign has blossomed into quite a program.

He does only about thirty minutes of calisthenics a week ("Am I bored? Of course! It's like taking medicine"), but he does them regularly, usually just before going to bed: running in place, raising legs, "bicycling" while lying on his back.

He also owns a real bicycle, and uses it once or twice a week. When he does, he is likely to ride for five or ten miles, and he always makes a special effort to give his heart the most arduous possible workout on the up-side of hills—a practice that is decidedly *not* recommended for anybody who is not in superb condition.

Between three and five times a week he walks for about an hour in his neighborhood. "It's a marvelous luxury to be able to be alone, to think, to enjoy the pleasure of breathing," he said. "There are no phone calls. I enjoy the foliage and the city. What a kindness to oneself! The truth is those 'lost' minutes don't make a damned bit of difference."

Two or three times a week the doctor also walks to and from the hospital, a distance of 1.8 miles each way, and he always tries to walk at a pace that he has clocked with a pedometer at 5.2 miles per hour (about 2.5 m.p.h. is normal).

Does he walk rain or shine? "Of course, there's nothing like walking in the rain!"

Does he walk in snow and ice? "We have clothes and boots!"

Dr. Hellerstein walks a great deal in the hospital, and some of this exercise, too, is voluntary. His office is located 136 paces away from his secretary's desk, but the doctor has never tried to make the arrangement more convenient. On the contrary, he welcomes the inconvenience as a blessing. It's part of what has become gospel to him, even though it sounds almost un-American. As usual, his phrasing is uncompromising:

"If I have the choice of doing something the hard way or the easy way, I'll do it the hard way."

Dr. Hellerstein is capable of being quite literal about enforcing this rule upon himself. Unlike some of his colleagues, he does not merely shun elevators for the distance of a few floors. His hospital is a six-story structure (seven, counting the basement), and the doctor is delighted when he gets a legitimate opportunity to bound up six or even seven flights of stairs at top speed. He has clocked his time for a six-floor sprint at anywhere between forty-five and fifty seconds, and he is at a loss to understand why more people insist on taking expensive trips to mountain areas to enjoy the therapeutic aspects of mountain climbing. He points out that most of us live around tall buildings that are superb mountain substitutes.

"We have mountains right in front of us," he said, beaming.

Dr. Hellerstein is not only managing to survive the rigors of his philosophy without a bit of trouble, but he is thriving on it. His blood cholesterol level is 220 (he has it checked every year and a half), and his general physical condition is so obviously superior that he must be the darling of his life insurance company. In the matter of diet, however, his body rebelled when he tried to restrict his fat intake too severely.

As we have seen in the case of Dr. Bruce Taylor, the Evanston pathologist, it is possible for some people to cut down on fats so that these will account for only ten percent of the total caloric intake. But this is a very extreme step indeed. When Dr. Hellerstein tried to cut down to 25 percent fats, the desirable minimum recommended by the American Heart Association, he found that he just could not live entirely within his medical convictions. "It was too stringent," he said. "At least it was for me. I had trouble with my bowels, especially constipation. I also experienced some depression." He estimates that he now eats about 32 percent fats, which still is drastically less than the typical American (about 41 percent fats).

To achieve this, the doctor's personal anti-fat crusade, initiated with his early reading about fats in the 1940's, had to be refined further. About twice a week

he sits down to a non-meat, non-fish, non-poultry dinner, perhaps spaghetti and a salad. His baked potatoes
are usually decorated with low-fat farmer's cheese.
Then, in 1952, he stopped drinking regular milk. True,
milk can be an important source of calcium, even for
adults, but Dr. Hellerstein believes that three or four
glasses of skim milk per week are sufficient for him.
Of his children, who range in age from three and a
half to fourteen, two are drinking skim milk and four
are on whole milk ("depending on need"). The Hellersteins are careful, however, to make sure that milk
does not play a large part in their total diet at any
age because they know how readily childhood habits
are carried over to adult life.

"Feeding children a quart of milk a day is absolute
nonsense," the doctor said.

In order to keep his weight down Dr. Hellerstein
weighs himself five or six times a week and watches
the size of his portions with the same intensity that he
brings to everything else he does. "I can gain weight
very easily," he said, "especially when I have to go to
dinners and banquets a lot. It creeps up. I could very
easily be a hundred eighty pounds very quickly. I'm
constantly denying myself. I put the brakes on right
away, whenever it's necessary."

His typical breakfast consists of applesauce or
peaches or pears, one or two slices of toast with peanut

butter, jelly or jam, coffee and, about twice a week, dry cereal with skim milk. On Sundays the Hellersteins usually have waffles, but Mrs. Hellerstein makes two eggs stretch for enough waffles to satisfy all eight members of the family.

For his lunches at the hospital the doctor may have a fish sandwich or a salad or, occasionally, a Canadian bacon sandwich (Canadian bacon is not nearly as fatty as the regular kind). Sometimes, when he is exceptionally busy, he may just nibble on a large peanut bar as he makes his rounds. The more or less traditional American businessman's lunch is scorned by him as "the height of asininity." It amounts to infinitely too great a caloric load in relation to the energy output of a male white-collar worker. ("We're not truck drivers!")

If Dr. Hellerstein must attend a banquet for professional reasons, he is careful to resist temptation. He does not touch the rolls and butter. He does not eat the full serving of the main course. And he usually has only one-fourth of the dessert. Quite possibly, his caloric sales resistance has been stiffened over the years by his low opinion of everyone who cannot control himself as neatly as he does. "Just because they're gluttons, you don't have to be," he said.

On special occasions, like everyone else, the doctor is happy to relent— but not much. What about when he takes his wife out to dinner? "Yes, we have chocolate cake," he acknowledged. "But we'll split one serving between the two of us."

When it comes to having dinner at home, the portions would strike most Americans as remarkable. One and a half pounds of ground chuck or round steak make enough hamburgers for eight. Two pounds will make enough meat loaf, with some left over for sandwiches. A rolled beef roast weighing between three and four pounds also is enough for dinner and some sandwiches. Three or four chicken breasts plus six chicken legs add up to a chicken dinner, with enough scraps left for another dinner of chicken chow mein.

How do the children manage on so relatively little food? We can only conclude that it must be mostly habit. At any rate, the male member of this reporting team visited the large old Hellerstein home on a wide, tree-lined street in the Cleveland suburbs and watched the youngsters at their evening meal. It was the same noisy, highly informal scene so familiar to every parent; everybody seemed to be healthy and happy, and there were certainly no symptoms of starvation in evidence. "No issue is made of food with the children," the doctor said later. "If they don't want to eat, nobody stands over them and says, 'Eat, eat!' They see Daddy doesn't eat eggs and their mother doesn't eat eggs, but nobody says, 'Don't eat this or that.' "

Guests also are not regimented in the Hellerstein home. At dinner parties the servings are what Dr. Hellerstein describes as "modest," but seconds are readily available, and there is quite likely to be a chocolate icebox pudding with lady fingers and "a little" whipped cream for dessert or perhaps brownies and sherbet. Comments on healthy eating habits are taboo on such occasions. "I abhor the boor who'll spoil food by imposing his ideas on his guests or hosts," the doctor said. However, since he believes that Americans eat far more salt than is good for their blood pressure, there has been no salt shaker on the Hellerstein table since sometime in the 1950's. "It's an insult to the cook," the doctor observed.

The "cook" in his home is a busy one. Dr. Mary Hellerstein usually works only one afternoon a week (at a pediatric clinic) and, at the age of forty-four, this small, quiet, surprisingly girlish-appearing wife does have a weight problem. She is five feet seven inches tall, weighs 145 pounds and has at times weighed as much as 150. "I would like to be a hundred thirty," she said. "It's hard for me. It's much easier when you're working full time." With so many children around the house, it seems to her that she is almost never anywhere but in the kitchen, fixing meals. The temptation to nibble is great and not always resistible.

"I try to eat fruit—mostly," she said, with a small, slightly embarrassed laugh.

Twice a week Mrs. Hellerstein goes to an exercise class ("the group helps"). She is active in the P.T.A. She serves on a local board of the Girl Scouts. Otherwise her physical activity is limited to the chores of an unusually busy housewife, and her husband concedes that this is quite enough.

"The average housewife uses as much, or more, energy as the average factory worker in a skilled or semiskilled job," he said. "And she doesn't have the rest periods or the short hours."

He is reasonably satisfied with the degree of his children's involvement in athletics, and any time he is taken by the notion that perhaps they've been too inactive for a while, he knows just the remedy. He takes them on a bicycle outing or shouts, "Come on, let's run the dog around the block." The distance, as the doctor has carefully clocked, is eight-tenths of a mile —nothing too strenuous, but nothing to be minimized when you've really decided to take the business of preventing heart disease seriously.

When will the rest of us fall in with this kind of life? Dr. Hellerstein recognizes that it's up to the doctors to lead the way, and as he watches his colleagues in his hospital, his ever-bubbling optimism gets a lift.

"The stairs are getting crowded now," he noted. "More interesting things are happening to the silhouettes of the cardiologists all the time. . . ." To him, the active way of life for all of us is just around the nearest street corner.

15

DR. BERMAN : *The Reluctant Revolutionary*

The majority of the doctors whom we interviewed are deeply involved in some of the most advanced diet research projects that have influenced medical thinking in recent years. Dr. Reuben Berman of Minneapolis, a wavy-haired, ever-smiling ultra-mobile and talkative man of fifty-eight, has different interests. At the time of our interview he was president of the Minnesota Heart Association. But mostly—indeed, practically around the clock—he is busy with his own patients. He is an internist and cardiologist, a clinical professor of medicine at the University of Minnesota. He practices in his office and at three busy hospitals every day. He is a warm, gentle man, but his work and temperament rarely allow him to sit still, and he likes it that way.

Dr. Berman, like all practicing physicians, is more readily influenced by the practical considerations within his environment than the men who live the researchers' more cloistered lives, and this is probably why he is frankly more reluctant to advocate change. "I know butter industries that are going broke right around me," he said. "If we all go to a diet of twenty-five to thirty percent fat, it means a complete change in our agriculture. I'm not prepared for it."

The doctor estimates that 40 percent of his own calories still come from fats. He says he has no guilty conscience about it, and for good reason. He weighs 175 pounds, the same as a decade ago (he is five feet eight) and his cholesterol level is 225, the same as it was when he checked it five years ago. He still uses butter, ice cream, pie and potato chips, and his family, which includes his wife, a former school psychologist, and six children, uses up about a pound of rather fatty kosher sausage a week.

How does Dr. Berman stay reasonably trim?

In a word, he just doesn't eat much. And while he

does sometimes crave food, he is usually much too busy to notice.

Dr. Berman is one of the doctors in our survey who eats no breakfast at all. He rushes off from his pleasant lakefront home shortly after getting up at 7 A.M., and when he arrives at his first hospital of the day, he has one or two of the six cups of coffee that he drinks daily. Ten years ago he had his coffee with cream and sugar; now, for caloric reasons, he takes it black. At lunch he has a conventional meat-and-vegetable meal, but no dessert. During the afternoon he may have a bottle of soda pop, but he does not bother to get the diet cola variety. Before dinner he has his one drink of the day: a martini. At dinner he does use butter on bread, potatoes and corn, but "very sparingly." He uses no margarine. He drinks ordinary milk, but has cut down from a glass a day to a glass every three days or so. He has reduced his beef consumption "somewhat," and his wife, Isabel, gets "economy" or "good" cuts rather than "choice."

"She tenderizes it by cooking hell out of it," the doctor said approvingly.

There now are four persons left in the Berman home, and they get along nicely on two pounds of pot roast. Their fish consumption has not increased, although Dr. Berman reported, "When I'm out for dinner now, I'll order fish instead of steak." He introduced this change about ten years ago. At about the same time he reduced his egg consumption from three to one a week. Since he is not a breakfast eater, this was not much of a sacrifice.

Dr. Berman is frankly interested in food. Twice a year he even bakes bread ("I like to *do* things"). But, perhaps because he must constantly teach heart patients to discipline themselves, he has learned to discipline himself with enviable fortitude. A large bag of potato chips lasts about a month at his house. And the doctor's bedtime snack may consist of nothing but a carrot. When he has cookies instead, as he frequently does, he has plain ones, and only one or two—never, but never, as many as three.

The doctor enjoys bowling, but he rarely gets around to it or to any other form of exercise except his incessant rushing about. He doesn't miss manufactured activity. "I'm too bushed," he said very happily. And since he estimates that his food adds up to no more than an average of around two thousand calories a day, it isn't hard to see why he is reluctant to turn his back on Minnesota's dairy economy and to undertake drastic changes in his fat intake.

Mrs. Berman, who is fifty-five, five feet one-half inch, weighs only 115 pounds and has never weighed more than 120. "I've never been a large eater," she said. "I come from a family that just doesn't seem to gain weight." She breakfasts on coffee and a slice of buttered toast. At about 10 A.M. she usually has more coffee and some fruit. Her lunches are conventional but small. Her alcohol consumption is just about nil, and her bedtime snack consists of a glass of tea with half a teaspoon of sugar. Once a week she may have a sandwich. And as long as the weather is not too snowy or icy, she invariably spends forty-five minutes a day bicycling around the lake.

The Bermans have one grown daughter who has had a weight problem ("She diets all day and then eats all night," said her father), but on the whole their attitude toward the eating habits of their children has been "permissive" and successful. Candy? "Some of the kids like it, some don't." Otherwise, the Bermans' efforts at food education have been limited to a single simple measure: They have always dished out small portions.

Obviously, in a busy family without special hereditary or other heart disease risks, it is possible to hold down weight without taking any steps but a single one: keeping calorie intake in balance with calorie output. But even the reluctant Dr. Berman wondered whether a special hold-down on fats might not be advisable for the typical American eater, after all. He seemed to be beginning to think of this as inevitable. "We may be facing a revolution," he said.

16

DR. HARRIS : *Feeling Guilty*

Dr. Philip Harris was one of the very few diet experts whom we met in the course of preparing this survey who considered it somewhat embarrassing to disclose his eating and exercise habits. Not that he was reluctant to delve into details. He simply felt that he was more firmly set in his ways than he ought to be, that he should have been making more changes in his habits over the years, that he wished he could, that it would be better for him and his family if he did. In a word, he thought he was doing his best, given his tastes and the pressures of his environment and job. But he was anxious not to have us hold him up as a nutritional model.

Dr. Harris is director of nutrition for the Food and Drug Administration in Washington, and it clearly pained him to confess that he gets very little exercise indeed. "I feel guilty about it," he said. "A good, brisk daily walk of two or three miles would be very beneficial. I just don't have the time, and I don't have the willpower to get up early enough to do calisthenics." And when we talked about his lunches in the government cafeteria where he normally takes his midday meals, Dr. Harris—a reserved, bespectacled man with an accommodating but distinctly professorial manner —reddened like a schoolboy when he confessed that he usually has pie for dessert about every other day.

We hasten to point out that we are not dwelling on Dr. Harris' "sins" in order to embarrass him further. We do so because the doctor and his family have actually readjusted their food patterns considerably more than most Americans. And if *they* insist that they have reason to feel guilty, perhaps the rest of us deserve to run about with faces permanently crimson to show our shame.

The fact is that Dr. Harris, fifty-six, and six feet two, weighed 180 pounds after World War II (his all-time record), but has not weighed more than 165 for many years now. He weighs himself "almost daily."

His blood cholesterol level is a close-to-normal 240, and he has it checked regularly once a year. His dietary changes have been substantial: A little over five years ago, he estimates, about 42 percent of his calories came from fats; now he lives on a 30 percent fat diet, a considerably more "modern" figure than the percentages reported by some of our other doctor-informants.

Dr. Harris' food switches came about gradually and over a long period. He stopped taking cream and sugar in coffee more than twenty years ago, but most of the major changes were made beginning about 1955. In those days he was using butter freely as a table spread, and his wife, Flora, a former social worker, used it routinely for cooking. Now Dr. Harris uses "almost nothing" to spread on bread, and Mrs. Harris uses Teflon pans and small quantities of margarine for cooking. Butter is in the house only for fresh corn in season.

"I like the taste of fat," Dr. Harris admitted with another one of his slow, guilty smiles, and it was not easy for him to become strict with himself about trimming visible fat off meats and switching from ice cream to sherbet. However, he took both of these steps early during his campaign to hold down on fats, and he has stuck with the changes.

A decade or so ago Dr. Harris enjoyed French fried

potatoes and peanuts, and he was terribly fond of doughnuts. All three items are only a memory now. And he has cut down "drastically" on his milk consumption, which used to be a quart a day.

Back in the 1950's the doctor was accustomed to the traditional American breakfast of two eggs every day, fried or scrambled in butter, often accompanied by bacon. Gradually he cut down to one egg a day, scrambled without fat in a Teflon pan. More recently he effected a further reduction to four eggs per week. His entire family, however, likes bacon so much that he has cut down on this high-fat food only "slightly." Mrs. Harris did purchase an elaborate two-level pan that turns bacon about as crisp as it can be turned without causing it to disappear entirely.

Cheese is another story. "We all love cheese," said Dr. Harris. "We have it in the house all the time and use it for cooking and snacks." Nor have the Harrises tried—like so many other cheese fanciers among our diet authorities—to switch their allegiance to cottage cheese or other low-fat varieties. They're just not willing to compromise their taste that much.

Cereal with honey (which Dr. Harris prefers to sugar for taste reasons) has become the mainstay of the doctor's breakfast. His luncheons are entirely conventional, although it turns out that his pie-eating is not as fattening as it sounds: He concentrates on the pie fillings and almost never eats the truly calorie-rich part—the crust. He does not usually snack at all except on rare occasions at bedtime; when he does have a snack then, it's always cold cereal, graham crackers and milk.

Dinners at the Harris town house, which is located in a newly redeveloped section of lovely old homes near Capitol Hill, tend to be traditional. Fish is served once a week. So is steak, although Mrs. Harris began several years ago to shop for cheaper (and therefore leaner) cuts. Chicken is on the table at least six times per month. There is no bread and butter with dinner except when company comes. This is also the only time when there is gravy or butter on the vegetables.

Until fairly recently the Harrises had a chopped-meat dish at the evening meal about six times a month, but Dr. Harris has been trying to cut down on the frequency. "You can never depend on it [the fat content] in the store," he said, "and besides, we might as well have some good meat to chew for ourselves." When the family does have meat loaf—still a favorite—three pounds of meat are ample for two meals plus about two sandwiches.

Like most lean-waisted doctors who do not eat a particularly restrictive diet, Dr. Harris does not happen to crave the calories that come in alcoholic drinks. These are the calories that he can afford to "invest" in pie and cakes, which he eats not only for lunch but also fairly often as dinner dessert. Nowadays Dr. Harris takes an average of only two cocktails a week, which is considerably less than the intake of most doctors we interviewed—except for the several near-tee-totalers. "I used to drink more," Dr. Harris said, "but as I got older I couldn't seem to tolerate it."

Mrs. Harris eats much like her husband, although she is not quite so careful about eggs and fats. She is in her fifties, five feet five inches tall, and has weighed as much as 125 pounds. For more than fifteen years, however, her weight has remained steady at 115 pounds. The two older Harris sons, twenty-eight and twenty-nine, have had no weight problems. The youngest, Philip Scott, sixteen, grew to be twenty pounds overweight not too long ago, but he managed to take off the excess poundage during a summer at camp where his counselor was an exercise-conscious former paratrooper, and the extra weight has not returned.

"Women are prone to overfeed their children," said Mrs. Harris with a knowing look. "Mothers are just trying to be too good to them. It's always, 'You're a growing boy, have another piece of this.'"

Clearly, the Harrises are a family for whom mild guilt feelings have paid off rather well.

17

DR. "SMITH" : *How To Succeed at Dieting Without Really Thinking*

When we confronted this doctor, who preferred to remain anonymous, with the same basic questionnaire that was answered by 65 other scientific authorities on dieting, the results were surprising. For example, we asked, "Have you become more careful in recent years to remove all visible fats from meats?" The doctor replied, "No." Our inquiries about recent changes in his consumption of beef, whole milk, bacon, butter, snack foods and other high-fat items also were answered by "No" or were not answered at all.

We knew that this physician had been an unusually respected New York practitioner specializing in metabolic diseases, diabetes and obesity. He had written a large number of authoritative scientific papers. His listing in *Who's Who* of affiliations, honors and offices held in medical societies was long and distinguished. At sixty-one, he was living in partial retirement on his farm but worked three days a week for a government agency in Washington, where he deals with nutrition problems of military personnel, including astronauts, and health problems affecting underdeveloped countries.

Was it possible that this doctor had decided to ignore the progress in his own specialty?

His note to us, enclosed with the questionnaire, was not conclusive. "I maintain that I do not have to watch my weight in the sense of the word that you use it," he said. "I eat a diet that satisfies my requirements for the conditions under which I live and work. This is what I call normal eating and requires no particular watching on my part. In other words, I am willing to admit that my choice of foods is undoubtedly *unconsciously* controlled by my many years of work in the field of nutrition, but I do not have to make any *conscious* effort to achieve what I consider normal eating."

When the doctor and his wife were interviewed in their exquisitely appointed apartment in a Washington hotel, the mystery soon evaporated. The doctor turned out to be an exceptionally dignified and somewhat crusty personality, splendidly tailored, slow-spoken, with close-cropped snowy white hair—the very picture of an eminent medical authority conditioned by decades spent in the presence of patients who strained to hear and weigh his every word. At sixty-one, he was five feet ten inches tall and weighed 152 pounds. He had weighed the same five years before, had never weighed more than 160, and had never had a blood cholesterol level higher than 220.

As the doctor was questioned about his apparent resistance to some of the questions in our questionnaire, it quickly developed that his reaction was simply that of a pioneer who was slightly annoyed at the fuss over matters that he had understood and accepted ages ago and had long since made a routine part of his life.

The reason the doctor had not cut down his butter consumption "in recent years," as our questionnaire had suggested, was that he stopped using butter in the early 1930's. It was also at about that time that he stopped eating his favorite cheeses, Brie and Roquefort, and switched to low-fat cheeses. He also stopped using sugar then. He had never eaten desserts except some occasional fruit or gelatin, so even thirty years ago he could hardly be expected to make changes in the dessert department. His exercise habits likewise date back to the same period: He found golf too time-consuming, but he always walked the two miles between home and office in good weather, he rode horseback, he walked a mile a day on hospital rounds, he enjoyed fishing and bird-shooting whenever he could, and he avoided elevators and taxis.

To this doctor it was quite obvious, even in the 1930's, that Americans, particularly the patients who came for treatment in his specialties, were eating too much fat and sugar and were not getting enough exercise. He decided early in his practice to watch his own habits, not only to protect his own health but as effective therapy for his patients and as an exercise in just plain honesty. "It gave me a feeling of confidence to talk to my patients without feeling like a hypocrite," he said. "How can I tell my diabetics not to use sugar? I would adhere basically to what I taught patients, so I could answer honestly when they asked, 'Do you do that?' " I wouldn't tell a patient to do something that I wouldn't do myself."

Over the years, then, a low-fat, low-sugar way of eating became second nature to the doctor, which really enabled him to stop thinking of it consciously as a dietary regimen. For practical purposes, it could be said that he never did eat ice cream; he had always eaten sherbet, and not too much of that. He had eaten skim-milk cottage cheese ever since it became available, mixing it with a little skim milk to make it more palatable; he could not really remember eating the regular creamed cottage cheese. And when he felt like nibbling something at night, he helped himself to a gumdrop.

In the early 1950's, when the first serious indictments of cholesterol and animal fats appeared in the medical literature, the doctor made further refinements in his habits. He had always liked fish, especially Nova Scotia smoked salmon with a little lemon, and so he ate more of it. In the past he had eaten about two eggs a week. By the mid-1950's he was down to two or three eggs a year. French fried potatoes? "I may taste *one* at lunch to remind myself how bad they are," the doctor announced. And as he began to look toward partial retirement, he decided to combine a healthy outdoor life with research into a nutrition problem that is of key significance to the typical American eater.

Americans are well-known for their love of beef. Beef is well-known, at least among nutrition experts, for its very high fat content—especially in the tastiest cuts. To change a major national meat-eating habit is a wearisome process; it may also be impossible. The doctor therefore decided to start a cattle farm where he would try to develop, through experiments in genetics, a new kind of tasty beef with a low fat content. It is work that requires time and determination. The doctor has much of both, and he would be too proud to admit failure, anyway.

Years ago, for example, he smoked three packs of cigarettes a day. When he decided to quit, he did not gain a pound, which is more than somewhat unusual for a very heavy smoker. "I was looking for it," he said, "but maybe because I was looking for it, it didn't occur."

The women in the doctor's family do not follow his rules quite so rigidly, but they, too, adopted his food patterns long ago and with fine results. The doctor has two daughters ("One is size eight, and the other size ten"), and his wife, at fifty-nine, weighs 135 pounds (she measures five feet four and a half inches). This doctor's wife eats much like her husband, although she does allow herself more eggs. Yet, when she shops, her market basket reflects a curious new double standard that is becoming more and more common in the homes of families who are sufficiently affluent to maintain live-in help.

She does buy butter. She does buy whole milk. She does buy ingredients for rich cakes. But these are for her household help. It is the kind of food that her servants, not yet eager to accept the lean ways of the best educated, most sophisticated eaters, insist upon. For herself and her husband, this wife studies the fine print on labels to find cheeses that are really low in fats. When she buys cookies, she gets the cheapest kind (usually oatmeal) because they tend to be the lowest in calories. And she buys generous supplies of vegetable oil because this is the basic fat she wants the cook to use when fruit pies or lemon sponge cakes are made for the doctor's guests (the doctor himself usually eats only the pie filling).

A typical dinner at this home is hardly a casual affair, even when the doctor and his wife are alone. "There's a feeling you're sitting down to a meal to which a great deal of attention has been paid," the doctor said. Considerable thought goes into the décor: the table setting, the linen, the proper color blending of the flowers. The service is flawless, and the food is good, if not very plentiful. Perhaps it is a case of eye appeal making up for stomach appeal. At any rate, this doctor and his wife are perfectly content. Theirs is the serenity of the wise and, yes, the righteous.

18

DR. HUNDLEY : *A Will of Iron—and a Stomach to Match*

None of the diet experts we have met thus far could be accused of being weak-willed. But it seems fair to say that none has quite displayed the iron will— and stomach—of Dr. James M. Hundley. His food habits are decidedly unconventional. He does not particularly recommend them to anybody else, and he is anxious to make clear that they do not reflect the dietary views of his employer, the United States Government. When this doctor was interviewed, he was the Assistant Surgeon General who dealt with nutrition problems in the office of the chief of the United States Public Health Service.* His habits, however, are interesting mostly because they are those of a man who does not want (and cannot afford) to be overweight, who does not want (and cannot afford) to appear critical of any major product of that influential gentleman, the American farmer, and who does have a weight problem.

Dr. Hundley (age: fifty-one; height: five feet ten) had his calories under control until he found himself in something of a trap early in 1964. He is another one of our doctor friends who appears calm and relaxed but is actually quite tense and under fairly constant pressure at his job. It is not astonishing, therefore, that he used to smoke more than two packs of cigarettes a day. Then he was named vice chairman of the Surgeon General's famous panel on smoking, the committee that finally rendered the official verdict that smoking and lung cancer are indeed related phenomena. So, in July 1963, Dr. Hundley gave up cigarettes and started smoking a pipe.

"I smoked it just like I smoked cigarettes," he recalled. "I inhaled and developed a heavy cough. One

---

* Dr. Hundley now is executive director of the Institute of Medical Sciences at the Presbyterian Medical Center in San Francisco.

Monday morning I inhaled the first couple of puffs and I couldn't catch my breath. It was as if I had the wind knocked out of me."

Dr. Hundley thereupon gave up smoking—and within six months his weight shot up from 160 to 177 pounds. Unlike most people who find themselves in such a situation, Dr. Hundley's choices were limited. As it happens, he had not eaten breakfast for more than twenty-five years. All he takes in the morning, except when he is traveling, is coffee with half a tea-spoon of real sugar and quite a lot of milk—the regular kind. ("I'm just not hungry when breakfast time comes.") Unlike many of his colleagues, he could not cut down substantially on eggs. ("I just don't happen to eat the meal where they serve eggs.") It was also against his policy and personal taste to eliminate such items as pork chops and cheese. Some years before, he had already cut down on pretzels, crackers and other snack foods that he greatly enjoyed, especially during his twice-a-month poker sessions with friends. ("Pop-corn was a big weakness of mine.") He had never had any desserts. ("I have no appetite for sweets. We don't have any desserts in the house; we don't even think about it.") So he could hardly cut down on desserts. And he quite understandably did not feel like giving up his relaxing two daily cocktails.

Clearly, Dr. Hundley's flexibility was unusually

limited. Yet he lost his seventeen excess pounds in about a year. Some of his adjustments were not difficult. For example, he switched from his favorite martinis to bourbon and water, thereby saving perhaps 50 or more calories per day. He cut down on coffee-and-milk, from ten cups to five per day. He limited bedtime food consumption to once a week, thereby drastically curtailing what he called his "fatal weakness" for cheese and crackers. What made the real difference was that he simply gave up lunch and subsisted on a single meal a day: dinner.

"Of course I was ravenously hungry later in the day and ate as much for dinner as I used to eat for lunch plus dinner," he reported. "But after about a week it was no problem." Dr. Hundley concedes that his training and his constitution no doubt permit him to function on a meal plan that might drive other dieters out of their minds. Twice during his previous career in nutrition research he managed to subsist for limited periods on water, coffee and tea alone. He found this was "no problem after the first day." With a gentle smile he added: "I'm sure I'm a little different physiologically."

The trouble was that even without breakfast and lunch Dr. Hundley found that he was not losing weight fast enough to suit himself, and so he took this occasion to step up his exercise substantially. He had always en-

joyed active weekends with such activities as horseback riding, hiking and ping-pong. But as he became
ever busier at the office, he no longer played tennis,
and he "never got around" to taking up golf, although
he frequently talked about it.

Instead of having lunch, therefore, he went for a
walk of one or three miles in downtown Washington.
If he had to attend a luncheon meeting, he walked
after dinner; that is, if he had dinner at all. The day
Dr. Hundley was interviewed for this survey, he had
enjoyed a large lunch (meat with gravy, dessert with
whipped cream), which was served, of all places, at
a large White House Conference on Health. So that
evening he planned to have just a little snack and his
usual drinks. This would come not only following his
usual walk but also a second new five-days-a-week exercise period: For thirty to forty minutes after dinnertime the doctor was doing calisthenics in the basement
with his twelve-year-old son, who was trying to get
in condition for his football team.

Dr. Hundley grew up on an Indiana dairy farm and
still uses butter, if not very much of it (there is rarely
bread and butter on the Hundley dinner table). He
also eats French fried potatoes, and his wife makes no
special attempts to get lean cuts of meat when there
is steak for dinner (four to six times a month). Nor
has he ever had his blood cholesterol level checked.

"I don't worry about my cholesterol if my weight is where it belongs. I don't believe cholesterol *per se* means a thing. If I were in a coronary-susceptible group, I'd feel differently. But my heredity is okay. We're not a coronary family."

Many diet specialists would take issue with some of Dr. Hundley's views and habits. They would undoubtedly feel that he tends to be immoderate in the way he practices moderation, that his methods of restricting his total food consumption place the system under needless stress. Yet his highly personal system works for Dr. Hundley, and he estimates that only about 20 percent of his 2,000 calories per day come from fats.

More significantly, his rigorous self-denials have served to alert his family to the dangers of overweight and prompted his wife and five children to cope successfully with weight management, each in his own way. His wife, who does usually have lunch and breakfast, eats sparingly enough to be somewhat underweight at 140 pounds. Of the children, only one ever had a weight problem: one of the doctor's daughters, who is now twenty-three and nicely trim. When she was sixteen, she was 15 pounds overweight. "We turned a little mild heat on," Dr. Hundley said. "We simply told her she was getting fat and needed to cut down. She just did it."

The Hundley children were kept busy with regular

assigned chores around their exurban Maryland home: washing cars and dishes, cleaning up the kitchen, raking the leaves around the homes of neighbors. Some years ago, chocolate "kisses" were replaced around the Hundley home by some much less fattening hard candies, and they were left in plain sight, to discourage sneaking. "The kids gobbled enormous quantities at first, but then they practically quit," the doctor said. "They probably just got bored." Ice cream is always available, but with a special touch. "The children have to go and get it," Dr. Hundley said. "It's not served. The kids have almost gotten out of the habit. Perhaps they'll take a cone before bedtime."

Another Hundley family technique is the weekend meal pattern. Mrs. Hundley fixes only dinner on Saturdays and Sundays. "The rest of the time the kids scrounge," the doctor said. "We eat only one real meal ourselves. My wife used to fix meals for them, but they stopped when they saw the parents were not eating."

19

DR. MUNVES : *Living It Up on Weekends*

Next to medical practitioners, nobody has been under more severe pressure about their personal weight management than the home economists, dietitians and public-health nurses who are supposed to teach the rest of us how to eat well and stay healthily lean, too. Not so long ago a great many women working as nutrition specialists were decidedly plump. Quite a few still are (so are quite a few doctors), but not nearly so many. It's been too many years since word got around that there really is no such thing as being fat and healthy at the same time.

As we have seen in the case of Dr. Helen Brown at the Cleveland Clinic, it is almost diabolically difficult for women who love food (and love to work with it) to watch their figures as closely as their doctor-bosses would like. But more and more of these ladies are managing more honorably these days—like Dr. Elizabeth Munves, an associate professor of nutrition at New York University.

Mrs. Munves, who is forty-five and five feet four inches tall, really is on the spot. She teaches home economists, dietitians and other professionals in the food field. She was president of the New York State Dietetic Association, served on the board of the *Journal of the American Dietetic Association,* and also functioned at N.Y.U. as nutritionist for the Student Health Services. She is married to a dentist and manages her home with not much outside help. She is raising two children, aged eleven and eight. Both of her parents have been overweight at some time in the past (which can make weight control extra difficult for hereditary reasons), and Mrs. Munves is frankly very fond of food.

She is not at all reluctant to confess, for instance, that going out to dinner once a week, usually on the weekend and preferably to a French or Armenian restaurant, is an outstanding high point in her busy life. "And when I go out for dinner, I eat anything," she said. "Vichyssoise and even frog's legs provencal." On weekends the Munves family also has wine for dinner (she has one glass, her husband two) and more liquor than the usual single daily cocktail. During an occasional very sociable weekend Mrs. Munves calculates that she may consume up to twelve hundred calories in liquor—a modest amount when compared to the intake of so-called hard-fisted drinkers, but quite a problem for someone who also likes food and is not particularly active.

Mrs. Munves also functions under some other handicaps. A plain-spoken red-haired extrovert who grew up in a rural area south of Ashtabula, Ohio, Mrs. Munves likes being among people, and her lament is familiar: "Any time you're going someplace, something is served to you." Like most housewives who enjoy cooking, she also prides herself on being a good hostess. She delights in serving chocolate mousse to her guests. And while she and her family almost never have bread or butter on the dinner table, both items are very much in evidence when there is company, and the bread will be hot and it will have been baked by the hostess.

As if these perfectly human preferences were not enough to wrestle with, Mrs. Munves has also been finding it increasingly difficult to do much about getting exercise. She used to play tennis and golf and enjoyed going for walks. And she still often swims, ice skates or bicycles with her family. But since the arrival of her children she finds herself so busy that she often does not finish dinner until 10 P.M., and a lot of her formerly free time is naturally devoted to the youngsters. She does avoid elevators when going up as high as four floors, and she sporadically tries to do calisthenics in the morning while listening to her French language records. She knows she should do the exercises more often, but as she put it: "It's a bore— as boring as watching paint dry. Besides, somebody has to get breakfast in the morning."

Nevertheless, when all this is said, Mrs. Munves weighed in at a trim 127 pounds at the time of our interviews, seven pounds more than she had weighed three years before, but ten pounds less than her top weight. "I'm fighting it constantly," she said, "and I figure I expend only about fourteen hundred calories a day." Yet even with all her formidable handicaps, hers is decidedly not a losing battle.

Her husband, Dr. Albert W. Munves, has had very similar problems, and since he became convinced a few years ago that recent nutrition research represents particularly urgent warning for sedentary middle-aged men, has made even more substantial changes in his eating and exercise habits—also with excellent results. At forty-seven he weighs 143 pounds (he is five feet seven inches tall). This compares with 155 pounds five years before and 160 while he was a dentist in the World War II army.

How does the Munves family account for these accomplishments in the face of their gourmet tastes, their hospitality and their weekend caloric splurges?

"We just don't eat as much food as we used to," said Mrs. Munves. In other words, they cut down during routine meals to save up for the special occasions, so that the *total* food consumption in the course of the week will be modest enough to keep their weights in balance or, if necessary, cause the weights to edge down.

At breakfast Mrs. Munves has juice, dry toast, black coffee without any sweetener, and an egg perhaps two to four times per week—always poached. For lunch she may have an open-faced cheese sandwich with a little butter ("I like the taste of butter, but I don't have much") or perhaps part of a can of soup. She suffers no hunger pangs in the afternoon ("If I were to smell somebody's dinner cooking, it would be different"). After her usual predinner martini the evening meal will be beef once a week or three times in two weeks, (usually chuck for steaks and bottom round for roasts, for cost reasons as well as the low fat content), chopped chuck as hamburger once a week, fish and poultry more than once a week, and occasionally another fairly lean meat like veal roast.

Most entrées are broiled in the Munves home, and there have been no French fries for more than a decade (partly because the family prefers baked potatoes or noodles). Bacon was eliminated more than five years ago ("empty calories"). Desserts are on the table perhaps twice a month ("I get to feeling guilty. I feel the kids ought to know what a pumpkin pie is"). This family does not care for salad dressings, so they eat salads raw with just a little salt. Mrs. Munves and her husband use skim milk for themselves for caloric reasons ("I don't think we've ever had whole milk"), but they have not switched from ice cream to sherbet, the caloric values being about the same. Mrs. Munves has ice cream at home about once a month—usually just one scoop at bedtime ("I just want a taste"). Normally she has no bedtime snack except some fruit. "Potato chips are my nemesis," she said, but ever since she was given a ninety-nine-cent bag while she was in the hospital and found herself gobbling the entire bag, she has been very careful to buy only small bags and only a few times a year.

If there is an additional "secret" in Mrs. Munves's successful control of hunger symptoms during her lean weekdays, it is probably her coffee consumption. "I don't function without coffee," she said, and on very busy days she has been known to drink as many as twenty cups. Many of our diet experts would consider this a quite unhealthy habit, but Mrs. Munves points apologetically to the fact that her workday lasts long into the night and also that she has never smoked. It is also relevant that any liquid can serve as an appetite depressant, particularly if taken in quantity.

Her husband found that he had to be even tougher with himself in order to bring down his weight and keep it down. He still has just a little touch of butter on one slice of breakfast toast, and he eats an egg five mornings a week. But ten years ago he began cutting down on his lunches by eating only one slice of the bread from his sandwich, and three years ago he went further: He has nothing but an eight-ounce cup of yogurt ("not for therapeutic but caloric and satiety reasons") plus one of the six to eight cups of black coffee that he drinks per day.

"Nighttime is my problem," said Dr. Munves. "Like my wife, I've never smoked. Black coffee is a good substitute, but you do get pangs. I think they're boredom pangs more than hunger pangs. I sometimes have a plain oatmeal cookie." Both he and Mrs. Munves have consciously cultivated the habit of eating much more slowly than they once did. "It's true," they said, "a little goes a lot farther that way." For caloric reasons Dr. Munves also switched five years ago from martinis to Scotch and water or gin with a low-calorie tonic mixer.

Unlike his wife, Dr. Munves said he had become "quite compulsive" in recent years in his efforts to be absolutely sure to get in a reasonable amount of physical activity every day. The walk between his Washington Square apartment house and the subway, and then from the subway to his office, adds up to about a mile for the round trip. Dr. Munves sturdily marches the full distance, no matter how bad the weather may be. He plays tennis once a week and performs twelve to fifteen minutes' worth of Canadian Air Force exercises every morning. "There has to be a *really* good reason to skip it," he said.

Food is just about never a subject for discussion in the Munves home, and it is certainly not an issue with the children. There simply aren't many "extras" around. Neither youngster ever had a weight problem. They normally eat ice cream once a day, at home or in school, and a snack at home does not mean having a sweet—it's more likely to be dried fruit, juice, whole milk, a pretzel or, once in a while, a sugarless candy substitute. On Sundays they share the family's "treat" breakfast of waffles or pancakes with maple syrup, but there are never any sugar doughnuts, jams or jellies, soda pop or cake icings. They have never, to their parents' knowledge, had a lollipop. Since their father is a dentist, they have, of course, heard that candy can cause dental problems. But even though they have not been lectured extensively on the subject, they have started bringing home candy from parties where they were expected to eat it. "We've brainwashed them, I guess," their father said, smiling.

20

DR. CHRISTAKIS : *Chief of the Prudent Dieters*

When Dr. Norman H. Jolliffe became ill in 1961 and decided to hire a new assistant, it was obvious to all concerned that the new man, whoever he would be, would have to agree to live on "The Prudent Diet" if he was going to do his job properly. Dr. Jolliffe was director of the Bureau of Nutrition in New York City's Department of Health at the time. He had designed the Prudent Diet for members of the department's "Anti-Coronary Club," a heart-disease prevention program that had already attracted national attention. The diet kept down fat to between 30 and 33 percent, much of it in vegetable rather than animal fats, and there were indications that it actually lowered heart-attack risks for the middle-aged male New Yorkers who belonged to the club.

Dr. George Christakis, then thirty-three years old, knew about the diet when he called on Dr. Jolliffe at Beth Israel Hospital to discuss the position. He immediately said he would not mind living on the Prudent regimen, and he got the job. "The diet made sense," he told us. "It took care of all the essential nutrients, and it introduced a sense of moderation with fats." About a year after Dr. Christakis went to work for Dr. Jolliffe, the first detailed reports from the Anti-Coronary Club showed conclusively, for the first time, that the diet evidently did save lives. Subsequent statistics, reflecting additional years of eating experience by the Anti-Coronary Clubbers, continued to strengthen the evidence, right up to the present time.

Dr. Christakis was delighted. "It was a nice fringe benefit of the job," he said.

When Dr. Christakis was interviewed at his suburban New Jersey home for this report Dr. Jolliffe had been dead for some years. Dr. Christakis had succeeded him.* The Prudent Diet was becoming increas-

---

* Dr. Christakis now is assistant dean of the Mount Sinai Medical School.

ingly popular with doctors and clinics throughout the country, its main attraction being that while it is, in fact, a therapeutic diet, it doesn't appear to be one to the average eater. No special foods are required. No unusually burdensome restrictions are imposed. Dr. Christakis, another of our spectacularly mobile, enthusiastic and youthful-looking interview subjects, expected to stay on the diet forever. His weight had ranged from 165 to 168 pounds before he went to work for Dr. Jolliffe (Dr. Christakis is five feet eleven and a half inches tall). Now it was down to 163. His blood cholesterol level, once at a comfortable 220, was down to an exemplary 190. Best of all, Dr. Christakis *felt* marvelous and relished the idea that he had reduced the risk of heart disease for himself and his family.

As it happened, the doctor had even less trouble getting used to Dr. Jolliffe's regimen than most new members of the Anti-Coronary Club. Dr. Christakis is of Greek extraction, and fish and vegetables had been staples in his diet since childhood. Even before 1961 he was eating fish as often as two or three times a week (including fish-sandwich lunches), and as far back as his days in Public School No. 54 he had won the applause of his teachers for being a boy who not only ate his spinach but was downright fond of it.

Yet in 1961 he was eating butter with meals. He was eating quite a lot of beef, including hamburgers (ground chuck) twice a week. He often had French-fried potatoes, and he ate quite a bit of cheese, especially Greek feta cheese. He normally had six to eight eggs a week, fried in butter. He was also partial to cinnamon buns, corn muffins and pie, especially apple pie. Much of his food was cooked in olive oil, according to Greek tradition. On the other hand, he did not care much for liquor. "I'm a poor drinker," he said, "although I've managed to learn to like vodka."

Under the rules of the Prudent Diet, the doctor switched from butter to margarine, and his wife, Emmy, who used to be a nursing supervisor at Presbyterian Hospital, began cooking and baking with corn oil and margarine. The doctor no longer touches French fried potatoes, he takes his baked potatoes dry and eats cheese only about twice a month and always as part of a meal. His desserts are normally limited to fruit. He eats four eggs a week—only at breakfast and either soft-boiled or hard-boiled, never scrambled or fried. He has cut down on beef (steak and hamburger once a week each) and eats no pork except for an occasional ham sandwich. Lamb, a very fatty meat that is popular in Greek cooking, is now reserved for festive occasions. The usual substitute in the Christakis home is chicken, and the doctor estimates that he has also about doubled his consumption of relatively lean veal. He had always been meticulous about removing visible fat from all meats. He likes liver, which contains considerable dietary cholesterol, but he now eats it only in restaurants and no more than once every two weeks or so.

Perhaps the most drastic change in the doctor's diet was the doubling of his fish consumption, which is a mainstay of the Prudent Diet because it substitutes polyunsaturated fats for saturated fats. Much of the increase came at lunchtime in the form of fish sandwiches or salads. Like many of our diet experts, Dr. Christakis is lucky in that he likes tuna-fish sandwiches, because he eats them with considerable regularity, along with sardine and tomato sandwiches, shrimp salad and sliced chicken or turkey sandwiches. He sometimes adds a little milk to his coffee, and though he uses skim milk for his breakfast cereal, he does not ask for skim milk in restaurants.

"When I'm eating with somebody, I don't like him to think I'm on a therapeutic diet," the doctor said. "I don't ask for corn oil for the salad, either. I don't want anybody to say I'm crazy. I'll just say, 'Easy on the Russian.' But I'll ask for double or even triple servings of lemon wedges for my fish."

Dinner at the Christakis home is a normal meal, although the portions are modest enough to save up some calories for the weekend. "I always leave myself open for one splurge on Saturday or Sunday," the doctor said. "There is an occupational hazard in ordering a nice Salisbury steak if you're being watched. But I assure people I've been eating fish four or five times that week, so it's okay to eat the steak."

His dinners at home emphasize fish, especially swordfish and charcoal shrimp, which are popular with the three Christakis boys, aged thirteen, eight and seven. There are no predinner cocktails, but twice or three times a week Dr. and Mrs. Christakis have either a glass of beer with their meals or about a glass and a half of chilled white Greek wine.

The doctor often works at his professional writing until 1 or 2 A.M., and he does get hungry during the evening. He usually manages to get along on an apple and perhaps a glass of milk. Very occasionally he will fix himself a tuna-fish sandwich or a bowl of corn flakes with some sugar, skim milk and perhaps half a banana.

Because of an interesting experience in his youth, Dr. Christakis is well aware of (and therefore able to guard against) emotional factors that cause him to overeat if he isn't careful. An unusually bright student, he was able to go through New York University in three years. The Columbia University Medical School refused to accept him unless he waited another year because school rules considered him too young. This caused him to feel extremely frustrated, and he proceeded to gobble up so much additional food that his weight shot up from 170 to 185 pounds in a matter of weeks. Fortunately, once he settled down for a year of graduate school, the newly acquired fifteen pounds were not hard to take off.

It was also in his youth that Dr. Christakis learned to appreciate extracurricular activities, especially the fact that a multiplicity of interests tends to keep people active, and active people who are rarely bored are almost never so preoccupied with food that they become fat. In high school he was the concertmaster in the school orchestra (he studied for ten years at the Juilliard School of Music and still plays the violin very well). He also fenced, played third base for the 103rd Street Sharks and played basketball up to the time he entered medical school. Nowadays he finds calisthenics too dull, but he is almost always too impatient to wait for elevators. Several times a week he climbs to a fifth-floor hospital clinic. "I'm ashamed to say that when I take two steps at a time, I arrive flushed and my heart pounds," he said, but he knows that rugged regular exertion helps to keep an already well-conditioned person's heart in shape.

When he went to work for the city health department in downtown New York he found a way to use his new location as the scene of some mild, pleasant exercise at least three or four times a week. He simply spent most of his lunch hour walking around the neighborhood inspecting interesting stores that sell boats, guns and other items that fascinate him.

"I love to get away and roam," he said.

Mrs. Christakis, who is small, dark-haired and quiet, finds herself forced to do considerable roaming herself, since she does all the housework in her three-level home, and her sons, John, Michael and Paul, require the usual formidable logistical support that is expected these days by all small suburban boys. Nevertheless, Emmy Christakis has fought overweight with only intermittent success ever since she stopped working in the hospital in 1956. "I enjoy my food," she said. "I watch myself, otherwise I'd weigh even more, but I'm overweight." She is forty, five feet three, weighs 139 pounds (compared with 131 in 1961) and worries about it.

She has also made changes in her eating patterns. She has stopped eating ice cream. She has cut out most between-meal nibbling except for apples, carrots and some yogurt occasionally late at night, and the inevitable "tasting" when she is baking bread with her Greek-born mother. Her egg consumption is down from the pre-Prudent Diet days, when she had eight or ten scrambled eggs a week, to four or five a week, always boiled. She has stopped buying commercially baked goods, but she does bake pies (with vegetable oils) once a month, as well as muffins or cupcakes perhaps once every two weeks (she fixes two dozen at a time.) Her alcohol intake is even more modest than her husband's. The main problem seems to be that it is difficult for Mrs. Christakis to cut down at suppertime.

"That's where everything adds up," she said, looking guilty.

It doesn't add up to all *that* much, however, because Mrs. Christakis, like most of the doctors' wives we interviewed, is a rather conservative shopper. One and a half pounds of ground chuck make enough hamburgers for herself and her four men. Four pounds of bottom or top round make plenty of pot roast, with leftovers. She buys no potato chips and gets cookies only rarely, but she shops for vegetables with great care, usually in New York's Ninth Avenue specialty vegetable markets. One of her favorite recipes is a casserole featuring artichoke hearts as the main ingredient; she adds small carrots, small potatoes, a little onion, oil, very little flour, a little water and some lemon juice.

"Sometimes I'll just cut up a million vegetables and bake them," she reported.

The three Christakis boys are active, but, like most of the doctors we interviewed, their father was fretting that they were not active enough for their own good. Like other doctors' children, however, the boys were not subjected to health lectures. "I don't like to make weight and nutrition an issue with the kids," Dr. Christakis said. "We don't propagandize the children." The boys have no weight problem. As infants, they were on a demand schedule. Later, and right up to the present, their milk was always mixed: half skim, half whole. They learned not to demand soda pop at home, and some time ago their mother stopped giving them snacks when they came home from school around 3:30 P.M., because they seemed to be getting "picky" at dinner.

"If you let a child get hungry before a meal, that child will eat anything," Mrs. Christakis said, smiling gently. She should know, because her children have even learned to like dandelion leaves with lemon and vegetable oil, in lieu of more conventional vegetables.

Dr. and Mrs. Christakis believe in informality and were delighted to open their refrigerator for inspection. We found it to be as full as the larder of any well-to-do American family, but there was also ample evidence that this couple has found a way to control what is undoubtedly the nation's principal dietary sin: excessive consumption of fats. In the Christakis refrigerator we did find a little margarine and mayonnaise. But we found heaps of vegetables and fresh fruit. *Way in the rear*, we uncovered a good-sized box of ice cream, but its appearance confirmed the doctor's testimony that it had been in the refrigerator for about two months. We also found a small can of chocolate syrup, but it must have been left there as a mere memory of things past. The syrup had congealed long ago.

21

DR. RINZLER : *Confessions of a Cake Eater*

In 1958 Dr. Seymour Rinzler went to work as cardiologist in charge of the Diet and Heart Disease Study in the Bureau of Nutrition of New York City's Department of Health. His blood cholesterol level then was 330. Recently it has been 226. Nobody can say with absolute precision how this change will ultimately affect Dr. Rinzler's lifespan. However, on the basis of heart-disease deaths found among people with high cholesterol levels (and 330 is very high), Dr. Rinzler gave us this prognosis: "I would say I am a minimal risk. Before, I would have had six times the chance I now have of having a heart attack."

It is important to appreciate that Dr. Rinzler faced his problem even though he was never overweight and therefore did not have to embark on what most of us would call "a diet." That is, he did not have to eat less. He did have to eat differently.

At 53, Dr. Rinzler, a calm, compact, gray-haired fellow with lively light-blue eyes, weighs 149 pounds (he is five feet six). He still fits nicely into the Eisenhower jacket that he wore overseas as an army heart specialist in World War II, and his top weight of 157 pounds, which he reached in the mid-1950's, was hardly cause for alarm.

When Dr. Rinzler joined Dr. Jolliffe in 1958 to help run the Health Department's Anti-Coronary Club, the club's now famous Prudent Diet was very much in the experimental stages. "We're all very smart now," said Dr. Rinzler, "but then we didn't know that if you ate in a certain way you could get your cholesterol down." So, for a while, Dr. Rinzler was asked to remain part of a control group of more or less normal eaters whose health was being studied so their condition could be compared to what was happening to the Prudent Dieters.

Dr. Rinzler was an ideal specimen for Dr. Jolliffe's control group. He had become interested in arteriosclerosis (hardening of the arteries) as far back as 1941. "I didn't know it was going to be a growth industry," he said, but, unhappily, this is exactly what it did become. Progress had been made in the *treatment* of the disease once people were known to be afflicted with it. In fact, just the year before he joined Dr. Jolliffe, Dr. Rinzler had published a medical book, *The Clinical Aspects of Arteriosclerosis.* Prevention of the disease—or at least slowing down its progress before it became a real problem in a patient—that was something else. Little was known about it, and manipulation of the diet as a preventive step was a new idea. It interested Dr. Rinzler because the Jolliffe group was zeroing in on fats as a culprit, and fats were a whopping part of his diet.

"I'm not a gourmet," Dr. Rinzler said. "I don't get bothered by the monotony of things." So for years in the 1940's the doctor lunched on tongue or corned beef sandwiches with butter, usually at a convenient delicatessen. After some years he changed restaurants and started lunching on Swiss or American cheese sandwiches. These were equally high in fat content, but, as the doctor recalled, "Once I got into the Swiss and American cheese business, that was it." For dinner, year after year, usually five or six times a week, he had roast beef or steak or hamburger—never eating so much as to cause a significant weight gain, but always enough to keep the fat content of his diet very high.

The doctor does not care for liquor except on very special sentimental occasions. He likes sherry and Dubonnet, and he's the sort who nurses along a glass of ginger ale at most cocktail parties, so he was not bothered by this source of extra calories that often troubles busy, middle-aged professional men. But he was very much a victim of his sweet tooth. Not that he nibbled candies or other such between-meals temptations; Dr. Rinzler is not the type. But he was severely addicted to desserts.

"Strawberry shortcake was my cup of tea," he recalled. "When we went to St. Moritz, it'd be nothing for us to make a whole meal out of all kinds of pastries." The doctor often had Danish pastry as dessert for dinner. He enjoyed ice-cream sodas. His regular bedtime snack was coffee and cake. And he also loved cheese, especially blue cheese, Camembert or Edam.

As we have seen, Dr. Rinzler did not really eat a lot of any of these high-fat foods, or else he would have gained weight quickly, so it would clearly be unfair to call him a glutton. But he estimates that perhaps 45 percent of his calories came from fat. Conceivably the fat content of his diet may have been even higher.

This, then, was the diet that the doctor kept eating after he went to work for the Anti-Coronary Club. As the months went by, his blood cholesterol level climbed higher and higher, until it reached the dangerous peak of 330. "I helped to prove an important point," he said. "If you're having beef and strawberry shortcake all the time, you can maintain your weight, but your cholesterol goes up." He recalled that he was frankly somewhat startled to see this happening in his own supposedly well-disciplined life, and he decided the time had come to do something about it. He did not have to "diet" in the sense of eating much less. He mostly had to eat less fat. And so he started eating according to the rules of the Prudent Diet and has been eating like his patients in the Anti-Coronary Club ever since.

"I'm taking my own medicine, but I believe it, too," he said.

The doctor had always breakfasted on orange juice, toast and coffee, so he had no eggs or other such high-fat breakfast habits as bacon to give up. For lunch he switched to tuna-fish sandwiches without butter. At dinnertime he cut back beef to two or three times a week and increased fish, veal, spaghetti and poultry consumption. He switched from butter to margarine and from French salad dressing to corn oil and vinegar. He still eats French fried potatoes occasionally, but they are prepared with vegetable oil. Ice-cream sodas, ice cream and sherbet he has decided to give up. "Cake is what I miss most," the doctor said, "but we have substitutes." Instead of his beloved strawberry shortcake and chocolate layer cake he now eats sponge cake and angel food cake, which are relatively low in fats. His wife, Rita, has even discovered a low-priced commercially baked fruit pie that is made without butter.

The doctor is not a fan of exercise ("I feel more peaceful not having to pick up golf clubs"), but he recognizes its importance and does his best. "I do purposeful walking," he said. Twice a day he walks his English springer spaniel about ten blocks. He also walks the eight blocks between his home and office, and he makes a point of walking "pretty fast."

Mrs. Rinzler, who is forty-eight, five feet one, dark-haired and vivacious, had a more acute problem than her husband. When she was interviewed for this survey, she weighed a model 112 pounds, which was pretty much her normal weight. However, one and one-half years previously she weighed 160. The enormous gain occurred because her physician, for reasons unrelated to nutrition and heart-disease problems, had placed her on a medication that happened to be weight-producing. The impact of the drug had sent her cholesterol level soaring to 300 (it has since come down to 220) and made dieting unusually difficult.

Mrs. Rinzler accomplished her weight loss under

medical supervision, but she credits much of her success to vanity ("I like to dress well") and to the Prudent Diet. To lose poundage, of course, she had to eat much less than her husband: a maximum of fourteen hundred calories a day compared with his "maintenance" quota that averaged about twenty-two hundred. And she finds comfort in some crutches: She still smokes two packs of cigarettes a day ("Recently I quit for four days; I thought I'd go mad!"). She fills up with an average of about four bottles of low-cal coffee soda a day. And instead of her usual snack of an apple around 9 P.M., she still cannot resist sometimes eating as many as four slices of toast with jam. But the fat content of her diet is drastically reduced, much like her husband's, and this was a major help in cutting down on calories.

Nowadays Mrs. Rinzler does not mind at all shopping for lean little seven- or eight-ounce minute steaks instead of sirloin, porterhouse or filets, and in the supermarket she always watches carefully while her chuck steak is being ground for hamburger, so she can be positive that all visible fat really has been trimmed off.

"We came at it from different angles and for different reasons," said Dr. Rinzler, "but it all adds up to the same thing."

The Rinzler children—Lois, who is twenty-five, and

Robert, twenty, who is studying at the University of Michigan—both have had some weight problems. But Robert took off his overweight at fourteen, when he wanted to make the school wrestling team. The daughter's weight has been normal since her marriage to a young physician. ("She was the one who ate her way through problems," her father said.) The elder Rinzlers were relaxed throughout it all. "I never forced the children to eat," said Mrs. Rinzler, "and I never forced them not to eat. One is just as bad as the other."

22

DR. SCHILLING : *Stopping Trouble Before It Starts*

Dr. Fred J. Schilling is a bear of a man: huge, big-boned, well tanned, with an enormous shock of gray hair, a booming voice and a way of conveying, almost the instant you meet him, that life is really pretty darned nice. To be specific, he is forty-nine, six feet three inches tall, and weighs a well-muscled 200 pounds. Dr. Schilling is an internist and medical director of the Continental Insurance Company, but he was interviewed at his Long Island home, where he also maintains a private practice as a consulting cardiologist. It's a home that seems tailor-made for him: three acres, thirteen rooms, seven baths and enough outside play equipment for a small summer camp— monkey bars, slides, ropes swinging out from trees, a tennis court and a handball court. The *pièce de résistance*, however, is the inside staircase. Along the paneled wall right next to the steps, in neatly ascending order according to age, hang color pictures of the doctor's children. Luckily, it's a long flight of stairs because there are eight Schilling youngsters, aged six to fourteen.

But these are externals. What's far more remarkable about the Schillings is that the entire family's food habits have been changed, drastically and permanently, beginning just a little over five years ago. The logistical problems were formidable, but Dr. Schilling is convinced that the operation is not only a success but that his children will thank him for it for the rest of their lives. Meanwhile, he lives with the satisfaction of knowing that he has done his professional (as well as fatherly) best to start preventing future heart trouble for his youngsters at a time when it will do the most good: early in youth, when eating patterns—so often difficult to change in later years—are first established.

Dr. Schilling is a careful, experienced medical researcher who is not in the habit of kidding himself, yet the results of his experience with his children exceed his expectations. "Their taste buds have changed," he reported. "Fat, rich ice cream has become repulsive to them. If they get whole milk served to them in a restaurant now, they actually detest it. They've reacted to skim milk like the fellow who didn't want to drink his first martini. Pretty soon he won't have anything else."

The reeducation of the eight little Schillings began shortly after Dr. Schilling started to reeducate himself. His company sells a lot of health insurance, and one principal goal of the doctor's job coincides with his own consuming passion in life: to develop new ways of preventing serious health problems before they ever start in the first place. His company has found that it's good business and benevolent employee relations to let Dr. Schilling propagandize its 12,500 staff members with the best techniques in preventive medicine that he can find as new research becomes available. Some years ago these duties prompted him to become interested in the New York City Health Department's Prudent Diet. He recalled how the death rate from coronary heart disease had dropped in Holland and elsewhere during World War II when the diet of the population, perforce, was greatly reduced in fats. The ideas of Drs. Jolliffe, Christakis and Rinzler consequently made good sense to him from the start. He then cooperated in some of the Anti-Coronary Club's research projects, became firmly convinced of the Prudent Diet's value and began teaching it to his company's employees.

"Prevention!" he boomed. "Prevention is what we've got to learn to practice in medicine, especially in heart disease. When you have to *treat* it, all too often you just become the assistant to the undertaker."

Once he had investigated the apparent effects of the Prudent Diet, Dr. Schilling found that he had to undertake radical changes in his own habits. He stopped eating butter and switched to margarine. He gave up his favorite food, ice cream, and switched to fruit ices, and he has even these only quite rarely now. He cut down his egg consumption to two per week; the eggs are still fried, as before, but they are now prepared with corn oil instead of butter. He cut down steak dinners from five per month to two and drastically increased his fish consumption. ("It's too bad so many women don't know how to cook fish.") Bacon is out. Whole milk is out; skim milk is in. Dr. Schilling is very fond of cheese and still eats it, but he rarely indulges this weakness between meals anymore.

"I used to have cheese as a snack," he said. "It was nothing for me to go to a good cheese store and drop five or six dollars. One day I just said to myself, 'Wait a minute, what am I doing here?'"

There were plenty of other long-standing habits that had to be broken, but the Schillings were resourceful in squeezing extra dividends out of their new way of eating. When the doctor laid down the law about increasing the number of fish dinners, he also purchased a boat. His freezer is now almost always loaded with family-caught fish. When the Schillings switched from whole milk to nonfat powdered solids (the family consumes three quarts a day), even the children got some satisfaction from watching their father's visible triumph over the resulting savings. The milkman used to collect $72 from the Schillings in an average month; recently the bill has averaged around $4.

As is evident from his own weight, Dr. Schilling is not one of those doctors who suffers more or less chronic hunger pangs. For breakfast he has V-8 juice, cold cereal with skim milk and just a little sugar, one or two pieces of rye bread with corn-oil margarine and three cups of coffee, usually with a little whole milk. He usually lunches in his office, normally just on a turkey, chicken or fish sandwich and coffee. Dr. Schilling does not snack between meals or at night, but his dinner portions are not stingy. It takes four pounds of ground chuck to fix enough hamburgers for the family and the maid.

Dr. Schilling is aware that he might be better off weighing under 200 pounds, but he feels that cutting down on fats is more important for him. "I'm comfortable at this weight," he said, and it has changed by only a few pounds in either direction in more than twenty years. The doctor usually enjoys two Scotches before dinner, but he has consciously decided to relax about fighting his relatively minor weight problem. "If I knocked off those two Scotches, I could get it down all right," he said, "but to me it just isn't worth it."

The doctor lives a tightly scheduled life, and the professional demands on his time run through the day as well as many evenings. Except for walking and stair-climbing, therefore, his exercise is largely limited to weekends. When Saturday finally rolls around, his activity is really something to be reckoned with. The Schillings have a yardman only once a week, and the work to be done around the grounds can be forbidding. In the fall the doctor has been known to rake leaves for a total of up to eight hours, and he estimates that he almost never spends less than sixteen hours a week functioning as his own maintenance man. Whenever he spends a full day working outside, he treats himself to a quart of beer.

The doctor's wife, Betty, an energetic, red-haired former nurse, is convinced that the medical thinking behind the changes in her family's food patterns is sound, and has changed her eating habits so that she now eats like her husband. Somehow, like most mothers of large families, she manages to be reasonably relaxed about it all, but she never lets the children forget the ground rules—or who is around to enforce them. Since Mrs. Schilling must take a drug that tends to be weight-producing, she does have a waistline problem herself. It is well under control, however: Betty is thirty-eight, five feet four and a half inches tall and weighs 128 pounds, her all-time top weight.

Her six girls and two boys don't leave her much time to brood about her figure problem. Even though she does have a full-time maid, Mrs. Schilling is rarely away from the kitchen. "It's like running a small restaurant," her husband said.

Food still gets fried in the Schilling establishment, but only with vegetable oil and only once or twice a week, with French fries as a special treat about once every couple of months. The potato chips are also made with corn oil, and the cookies are homemade and plain ("They're gone before they're cool"). Dry crackers are frequent cookie substitutes, and treats are dished out carefully by Mrs. Schilling and only at certain approved times. "I see mothers opening cookies for their children right in the store," she said disdainfully, "and I suspect that sometimes they only want them because they've seen them in a TV commercial." Since egg-salad sandwiches are frequently served at school for lunch, eggs are only for weekends, and there is never more than one egg at a time for each child.

Soda pop is also for weekends only ("There may be a bottle of ginger ale missing in the refrigerator occasionally, but there are no wholesale raids"). Instead of ice cream, there usually are popsicles or fruit ices. Mrs. Schilling bakes fruit pies with corn oil about three to five times a month, and once in a while there is pound cake, applesauce cake or another type without rich frostings or toppings.

Quite a bit of food comes into this house by the crate, especially apples and grapefruit. Six months before the Schillings were interviewed, they also purchased a case of chocolate bars. Much of the contents was still around, although all the children had lately had a bar as a special luncheon dessert instead of the usual plain cupcake.

Like so many of his colleagues, Dr. Schilling complains that his youngsters are not active enough to suit him. "We've practically got a park for them right here," he said. "These things are here to be used. I want the kids outside, but they're inclined to be lazy and follow the path of least resistance. I want them outside, and they do go, but it takes a lot of prodding."

It has been much less difficult to influence the youngsters against eating too many fats. Dr. Schilling, unlike most doctors whom we interviewed, pursues this point with his kids consciously, aggressively and systematically. "I tell them they're going to get their pipes rusty if they eat too much of this stuff," he said.

The lesson has sunk in, and Dr. Schilling is especially pleased when he can watch the evidence as the youngsters pick their food in restaurants. "You can't afford to take this mob out for dinner often," he said. "But they follow their new pattern when they do go out. They rarely pick steak and French fries, and they go for poultry and lobster and clams instead. Once in a while I do see them pick something with whipped cream."

23

DR. GLENN : *The Reform School that Gets Results*

Dr. Morton B. Glenn was the only one of our medical guinea pigs who conforms at least approximately to what the public calls a "diet doctor": He works with private patients who are overweight. He sees about one thousand of them a year, and about 80 percent of his practice on New York's East Side is devoted to treating obesity. Unlike many so-called diet doctors, however, Dr. Glenn was known to us as a well-trained internist who used to work for Dr. Norman Jolliffe of the New York Health Department. We knew that Dr.

Glenn was chief of obesity clinics at three hospitals, that his treatment was frequently so successful that even other doctors sometimes sent their wives to see him, that he rarely prescribed pills, and that he had the reputation of being a mighty tough cookie. In fact, from the stories we had heard of his patients, we had come to think of him as something of a reform school for dieters.

Long before we interviewed him, we also were aware that he was delighted with his reputation. We knew this because we had read his enormously successful book, *How to Get Thinner Once and for All* (Dutton), in which he copes with every weakness, weasel, dodge and excuse ever devised by weak-willed dieters. He wrote with evident relish: "Many of my patients dread facing me because they feel I am never satisfied with their performance and they are fearful that I will discharge them."

If you want to know how Dr. Glenn employs toughness as one of his tools to reeducate the eating habits of his patients (his sternness is by no means his only medicine), we suggest that you read his book. It's a good one. We're here only to tell you about himself and his family.

Frankly, we were disappointed. We had hoped to meet an ogre, but Dr. Glenn let us down badly. He is a gay little man with snapping blue eyes, a big smile, quick-darting body movements and fearful energy. He's another of these fantastically fit fellows (age: forty-five; height: five feet nine; weight: 150 pounds) who never sits still. He speaks rapidly, and for emphasis he likes to drum his hands lightly on the arm rests of his ever-swiveling office chair. It is next to impossible to imagine him asleep. His short hair is graying rapidly, but he looks easily eight or ten years younger than his age, and his enthusiasm for his work is somewhat overwhelming.

"I find it basically rewarding because the treatment of obesity can be a successful thing," he said cautiously. "Of course, I've got some real good failures, too."

Dr. Glenn has never weighed more than 165 pounds, and this was only briefly when he became bored during his days in the Navy in World War II and thought it would be "fun" to eat a lot and see how quickly his weight would go up. Once he found he could no longer fit into his clothes, he dieted his way back to 157 pounds in less than a month, simply by eating less. His civilian weight never exceeded 158 pounds, and his cholesterol level ranges between 220 and 250 (it used to be 285, which the doctor attributes to a family history of high cholesterol levels). The doctor weighs himself "almost every day" and says: "I'm constantly aware of my own weight."

Until 1959 Dr. Glenn nevertheless ate two eggs for breakfast every day and beef or lamb for dinner at least five nights out of seven. At that time, however, the trend of new research findings persuaded him to cut down drastically on animal fats. Now he limits himself to three "visible" eggs per week ("It was the most difficult change for me to make; for a long while I thought I couldn't survive on less than fourteen eggs a week"). He has pretty well given up orange juice for breakfast because of an allergy. So now he usually has several kinds of cold cereal mixed with modified skim milk or some toast and jam and margarine. He has not cut out bacon, but he admits, "I last had bacon about three months ago."

There's rarely more than ten minutes' time for lunch during Dr. Glenn's normally busy workday, and he usually eats in the office. His nurse may bring him a container of ordinary cottage cheese with a fresh hard roll, or a small can of salmon, a roll and a fresh tomato. He usually prefers to drink nothing. Often he eats lunch in his car en route to one of his clinics. On such days his favorite is a tongue sandwich on rye, with mustard but nothing else. Dinner isn't until 7:30 or 8 P.M., and the doctor confessed, "I get a little hungry, but it goes away."

Dinner is a normal meal, but beef and lamb have been cut down to twice a week, and fish, poultry and veal were substituted. Dr. Glenn considers bread and rolls one of his weaknesses, but there is no bread and butter on the dinner table. Steak will be on the menu once a week or once every ten days (more frequently during the summer cookout season), but the doctor's wife, Justine, still gets the best cuts. "I know it's wrong," she said, "but these are the facts of life. The lean cuts just aren't good." Dinner desserts are melon or half a grapefruit or dietetic gelatin— or pound cake "once in a blue moon."

"I thoroughly enjoy a drink," Dr. Glenn said, but the emphasis in this sentence belongs on the word "a." He happens to dislike Scotch. "Lately we've been on a vermouth Cassis kick," he said, "but in winter I usually have Canadian whisky on the rocks." Wine is served only when there is a dinner party or a major family celebration, and when there's wine, there are no cocktails beforehand.

The Glenns snack on ice milk during most of their evenings. The doctor's tranquilizer? "Television or medical literature," he said.

And yet, Dr. Glenn also told us, "I'm basically fussy about food. I adore French *haute cuisine*. I adore some of the French cream soups and quiche Lorraine with crab meat. I get very finicky about the way some sauces are prepared or how fresh a piece of liver is." When we questioned him, he confessed that his gourmet restaurant extravaganzas are confined to perhaps six occasions a year. Even then he orders fish nine times out of ten, never orders dessert and leaves a "moderate amount" of food on his plate.

"I have never been a plate cleaner," he said with pride.

Like so many men who are hyperenergetic and basically tense, Dr. Glenn smoked two and a half packs of cigarettes a day as recently as December 1963. For some time he had been convinced by the scientific research that shows cigarette smoking to be far worse than the vast majority of cases of overweight. Now the time had come when he was determined to do something about it himself. He gave up smoking, "cold turkey," gained about five pounds but did nothing about it for a month. Then, slowly, he cut down on his food and drinks to lose the five pounds again.

"I'm always aware of everything that goes into my mouth," he told us. "With my work, I can't *not* be aware of it. The trouble when I stopped smoking was that I had nothing to do with my hands. I didn't concern myself about it for a month because I first wanted to feel more secure about having given up the cigarettes."

On the problem of exercise, Dr. Glenn did not join his prevention-minded colleagues until the spring of 1967. We would want to be the last to diagnose that perhaps even a man like Dr. Glenn, who surely has heard every rationalization known to man from his patients, may have been rationalizing when he told us, "I've never been convinced that exercise is important to people's health." By 1967, however, he said he had been persuaded that exercise does have some bearing on the efficiency of the cardiovascular system.

So now Dr. Glenn does the Canadian Royal Air Force exercises for five to ten minutes each morning ("I put up with it without hating it"), and he reports that he "rarely" fails to perform this workout more often than one morning out of every ten. He has also started playing golf on Sundays and admits, somewhat grudgingly, that he has felt even better than ever since he began exercising systematically. He still finds it hard to prescribe exercise for his busy patients who are almost invariably engaged in sedentary endeavors.

"I've yet to find a patient who chops wood," the doctor observed.

Luckily for Dr. Glenn's professional and social standing, his wife, who is five feet five and one-half inches tall and weighs 118 pounds, has never weighed more than 125. Also, as a physician's daughter, she is blessed with a thorough background of caloric knowledge and a highly developed fashion sense.

"I simply love clothes," she told us, "and if they don't fit me, I push the panic button."

She even pushed the same button when her oldest daughter temporarily became fifteen pounds overweight at eighteen during a time when the girl was under some unusual tensions. Mrs. Glenn talked to the girl about it and promptly was lectured by her husband. "Leave her alone," Dr. Glenn said. "She'll be okay." And she was.

Mrs. Glenn now eats the same diet as her husband ("I used to eat just about an all-meat diet, mostly beef," she said). A dozen eggs will last this household for from two to two and a half weeks, and they're mostly for the children's friends. Two loaves of bread last for four days, and they're mostly for the maid. Hard cheese is for entertaining only. There is no butter in the house (just margarine), and skim milk has been substituted for whole milk.

"All of this would be very hard to do without a co-operative wife," said Dr. Glenn, with a fond smile at his spouse, and his hands beating out their drumbeat on his chair.

24

How Doctors Diet

It all boils down to this: The doctors who have changed their habits to take advantage of the latest lifesaving scientific findings *do* eat, drink and exercise very differently from most Americans, and so do their families, but nothing that these experts practice for their own health protection is particularly difficult to imitate by run-of-the-calorie dieters. In fact, you can live like the canniest, most up-to-date medical specialist simply by adapting the doctors' habits to your own accustomed ways.

We think this is astonishingly cheerful news, because these doctors, as a group, are unquestionably the most knowledgeable nutrition authorities in the world today. They don't merely read the books and scientific papers on diets and dieting. They write them. They run the laboratories where most of the current diet information and treatments used by other doctors originated in the first place. These are the doctors who serve on the nutrition committees of the U.S. Government and such organizations as the American Heart Association. They are the experts whose speeches at medical conventions you see reported in your newspapers. We talked with thirty of them in detail, usually at leisure in their homes; another sixty-six responded to our forty-four-part questionnaire. There were eighty-nine in all because seven interviewees also filled out the questionnaire.

As you have seen for yourself by now, they all turned out to be human.

For it's surprising but true that the experts are not ascetics or super-dieters. They shun almost no normal foods, and, by and large, probably eat a more varied fare than most of us. They don't count calories. They use no diet pills and no special diet foods. They don't give up most of their little personal food idiosyncrasies or cocktails. They don't constantly sermonize their wives and children about the evils of eating. Like the rest of us, some doctors are still trying to stop smoking but find that they miss their cigarettes or cigars too much and that they gain weight when they give up tobacco.

Above all, these experts are not forever "going on a diet" or struggling with their consciences because they feel they should. The chief reason for this phenomenon is an unusually interesting one. It illustrates one deep difference between the doctors and most of the rest of us. And while it seems to be, on first look, only a matter of semantics, it is actually basic. What we are talking about is the very meaning of the word "diet." To most of us, the word suggests a more or less drastically rigged reducing regimen that usually calls for the elimination of certain major foods and perhaps a considerable increase in the consumption of others —the whole business being supposedly guaranteed to turn the caloric tide in a matter of days or weeks, whereupon you may then feel free to go back to your accustomed ways.

To the doctors whom we interviewed, on the other hand, the most common use of the word "diet" suggests nothing of this kind at all. The "diet" that they themselves eat is their normal, everyday, year-in-year-out food pattern, and there is nothing temporary about it. This diet—what we call "The Doctors' Diet" —is by no means inflexible. In fact, as we have amply demonstrated in the preceding chapters, there is no *one* way to eat and exercise according to its rules.

There are as many ways as there are people and tastes conditioned by ethnic origins, childhood habits and the kind of human quirks that cause some people to grow weak at the thought of whipped cream while others think they might gladly commit violence for another handful of potato chips or a bagel with cream cheese.

This very flexibility, we believe, is one reason why the existence of a Doctors' Diet has remained unnoticed for so long. Perhaps it merely never struck anybody as being sufficiently different from normal eating to be worthy of the label "diet." As you have no doubt noted, however, there is no need to worry that the Doctors' Diet is ancient wisdom. It's new and different, all right. Its differences are just a great deal more subtle than what might be expected by a run-of-the-fad dieter who is accustomed to such gimmicks as lots of eggs or steaks or lots of liquor or perhaps no bread or other carbohydrates.

We are examining here, then, a truly sophisticated and modern no-formula diet. Some of its rules, as will become quickly apparent when we analyze the foregoing case histories in detail, are quite firm. Other yardsticks are still so controversial that even the experts whose views are reported here were in rather obvious disagreement among themselves. In a field where most of the important research is less than fifteen years old, this is as it should be. Moreover, you probably noticed that the differences among our authorities are relatively minor and will not make it any more difficult for you to use their personal food and exercise patterns.

We would caution you earnestly to examine these patterns in the light of common sense and to make no major adjustments in your own habits without your doctor's advice, particularly since your own health history may make it unwise to adopt certain changes that are perfectly acceptable in other cases. At the same time you can assume that the doctors cited in this study are highly qualified in their respective fields. They are not about to ruin their own health or that of their families with food and exercise habits that are of doubtful value. And you may also rest assured that these men and their families, just like you and us, regard eating as one of life's great gifts, a pleasure no more to be trifled with than well-informed prudence should dictate.

Of course, there were those few doctors who merely "eat to live" and never take a noontime break over anything but a tuna-fish sandwich without butter or mayonnaise. (One of them told us, "It would never occur to me to ask, 'What'll I have for lunch today?' ") But this is a tiny minority. Far more typical was Dr. Jeremiah Stamler, head of the Heart Disease Control

Section of the Chicago Board of Health, when he confessed, "I have to struggle all the time. I *love* to eat." And let's not forget that even Dr. Fredrick Stare, chairman of the Department of Nutrition at the Harvard University School of Public Health and one of the most zealous crusaders against caloric excesses, admitted wistfully: "I enjoy eating. . . . It would have been most pleasant to have had a couple of sausages and eggs for breakfast."

We're sure that you were also struck by the fact that most of our experts don't enjoy systematic exercising any more than most of us. Certainly their struggles to manufacture physical exertion for themselves sounded all too familiar, and so did the tone of their protests. At this point, just to comfort ourselves, it's worth recalling a few of these cries of anguish:

"I don't have the will power to get up early enough to do calisthenics." (Dr. Philip Harris, director of nutrition for the Food and Drug Administration.)

"The idea of doing jerk-ups would drive me nuts." (Dr. Ancel Keys, director of the Laboratory of Physiological Hygiene at the University of Minnesota.)

"It's as boring as watching paint dry." (Dr. Elizabeth Munves, associate professor of nutrition at New York University and former president of the New York State Dietetic Association.)

"Am I bored? Of course! It's like taking medicine."

(Dr. Herman Hellerstein, Western Reserve University.)

We venture to predict that by the time you finish this book you will be more than merely surprised by what these doctors are nevertheless able to do in order to live up to their scientific convictions. We hope that you have already developed a very definite feeling about these families. You may admire them for their ways. You may be somewhat awed by them. You may well decide that you don't wish to live as they do. Whatever your reaction is, we believe that we should share with you our growing conviction that the ways pursued by these doctors will pretty much be the ways of the future, whether we like it or not. To be sure, we will not all eat and exercise as they do. Not even all of our grandchildren will. But there is no question in our minds that more and more ordinary eaters are even now adopting more and more of these doctors' methods. Our common sense urges it. Our sense of self-preservation all but demands it. And if you, like us, have been on many "diets" and have lost and regained many pounds, again and again, you will probably conclude something else about the ground rules observed by these doctors: There really are no sensible alternatives.

All right, then, we have seen what the experts do besides denying themselves fried eggs and sausage on most mornings and managing, with notable exceptions, to put up with the ennui of man-made exercise. Now, what does it all add up to?

To begin with, and this is the No. 1 secret of the Doctors' Diet, *they are quite literally weight-watchers.* The weight of most of these doctors and their wives has remained remarkably steady over the years, and we suspect it's no coincidence that they climb on the scales far more often than most Americans. Most of the experts we talked to weighed themselves once or more a week. Of the sixty-six doctors who were surveyed by our questionnaire, forty-seven weighed themselves once or more weekly and fifteen weighed themselves each day. And they don't just examine the results with academic detachment. Whenever their weight creeps up a few pounds, they "put the brake on right away" and cut down on food or liquor or both. A gain of five pounds is considered positively alarming in these families.

Of course, it's not the mere act of weighing oneself that really counts; it's the application of instant fortitude in the face of an even slightly expanding waistline. You'll recall that Dr. Philip L. White, director of the Department of Foods and Nutrition of the American Medical Association, weighs himself only once every six weeks. Instead, he makes sure that he shaves with his undershirt off because his practiced eye tells him when his stomach shows signs of straining against his belt. When it does, he takes immediate steps. Instead of skim milk at coffee-break time (he switched from regular milk about eight years ago), he has a low-calorie soda. Instead of a bowl of soup with his luncheon sandwich, he has only a cup. At dinnertime he cuts down on portions. Dr. White's watchfulness at shaving time has paid off nicely. When we talked with him, he weighed 158 pounds. Five years before, he weighed 162; ten years previously 165.

Regretfully, Dr. White smoked two and a half packs of cigarettes a day and conceded that they served him not only as pacifiers but as appetite depressants, too. Smoking on such a scale is probably unique among our sample of experts, but giving in to one's weaknesses is not. It's just that most of the doctors are ingenious in devising ways to accommodate their quirks in moderate and medically commendable style. Remember how Dr. Irvine H. Page, senior consultant to the famous Cleveland Clinic and former president of the American Heart Association, smoked four cigarettes a day, but never lighted up the first one until the cocktail hour?

Dr. Page happened to have no trouble giving up his favorite food (peanut butter), but most of his fellow experts have not seen fit to make such sacrifices. On our questionnaire we asked, "What is your

greatest single food thrill or 'temptation'?" The re-
plies confirmed that eating for fun need not go out
of fashion, and that nothing in the human experience
is more subject to individual whim than the taste buds.
Of our 66 respondents, 46 confessed to at least one
caloric weakness. Among the dishes listed were ice
cream sundaes, apple pie, hors d'oeuvres, gumdrops,
chocolate, cheese, pastries, popcorn, and such headier
categories as "French gourmet dinners," "rich desserts," "any good food" and "my wife's cooking."

One lady doctor listed "whipped cream," but added
that she managed to ignore this craving. Others also
said that they tried their best to "avoid" their favorite
food. One doctor, who listed candy as his potential
downfall, said he kept consumption down by never
carrying change for his office building's candy ma-
chine. However, almost all others reported that they
did indeed partake of their forbidden fruit, but "in
moderation" or "with restraint." Typical was the report of Harvard's Dr. Stare that he is inordinately
fond of Liederkranz cheese with crackers. Typical,
too, was his wife's report that the doctor very rarely
eats Liederkranz, and the last time he had some he
nibbled on it so sparingly that she finally threw quite
a bit of it away.

Here we have isolated the second secret of the Doctors' Diet. This by no means exhausts the list of the

doctors' ground rules, and we will soon summarize how the country's most sophisticated eaters have managed to translate the latest scientific findings for themselves and their own families by changing their consumption of such specific foods as meat, eggs, table spreads and other staples. But before we do, it is crucial to understand how the doctors are able to apply a policy of moderation to all their eating and drinking. They have done it principally by redesigning at least two of their daily meals and all their between-meal snacks (yes, the experts do snack, as we have seen). Only dinner is likely to be a conventional affair. What we discovered simply is that *not one of our doctors (and few of their wives) eat what most of us approvingly call three "square" meals a day.*

The Doctors' Diet becomes most visible at breakfast, because that's the time when tradition is most apt to collide with modern medical thinking. Very few of our doctors had ever had problems with elevated blood cholesterol levels, and by no means all are convinced that cholesterol of itself is a life-shortening poison. However, all are acutely aware that eggs are the chief source of dietary cholesterol and that it's hardly a bright idea to pump quantities of this fatty substance into the arteries, where it might possibly help to trigger eventual heart attacks. Of the 66 experts who answered our questionnaire, 36 had cut down on eggs in recent years. The majority had also reduced their intake of those popular breakfast dishes that are not only high in animal fats (now suspect as possible factors in heart disease) but also rather rich in calories: thirty-eight use less butter; thirty-eight use less bacon; forty use less whole milk.

Among our other group, the doctors we met personally, the de-fattening of breakfast was an even more pronounced trend. Four of them had gone to extremes that are not generally recommended: They went to work on nothing but black coffee or coffee and juice. Many others enjoyed eggs or bacon only once or twice a week or only once a month or even less frequently. For these men, the once typical American breakfast had become a Sunday treat. The position taken by Cleveland's Dr. Hellerstein, the doctor who has eaten only one visible egg (eggs not used in cooking) a year since 1950, is still considered rather extreme, but there are more and more doctors who, like Chicago's Dr. Stamler have eggs once a month or even less often. And an increasing number of these experts now even remove the cholesterol-rich yolk from hard-boiled eggs whenever they spot it in a salad.

For many doctors, these self-imposed morning restrictions pose the day's touchiest dietary dilemma. Harvard's Dr. Stare posed the question succinctly when he asked: "What the hell are you going to *have?*" As we have seen, Dr. Stare cut way down on sausage and bacon. To cut calories further, he drinks only a little orange juice (two or three ounces compared with six or seven ounces some years ago). And, starting four years ago, he has been eating eggs only once or twice a month, normally when traveling on planes. His basic morning food (and that of many other doctors) is dry cereal. Luckily, Dr. Stare is fond of it and makes it somewhat more interesting by helping himself to about four different kinds and mixing them. Unlike many of his colleagues, he uses regular milk because even he finds skim milk tastes too much like water.

In addition to cereal, the doctors' breakfast leans mostly on coffee (often with skim milk and artificial sweetener) and toast with very little margarine or butter or, preferably, with jam or marmalade. It's worth keeping in mind how Dr. Benjamin Alexander, the hematologist at the Cornell University Medical School who gave up eggs nine years ago and stopped using table spreads about two years later, now prides himself on having injected a little variety into his mornings by keeping five or six kinds of jam to pick from. But the real answer to our doctors' morning problem is their principal appetite depressant, one that even the experts are rarely conscious of, and that is, in a word, work. The doctors' third diet secret is that they are notoriously *busy and very rarely bored*. The truth is that they normally don't have the time to think much about their appetites until the end of the day.

And a lucky thing it is, because almost none of the doctors we met had a "regular" lunch on a normal workday. Dr. Hellerstein put the matter pointedly when he told us: "We're not truck drivers!" We encountered several men who did find themselves ravenous by late morning and showed up in their hospital cafeterias for lunch rather promptly around 11:30 A.M. Most of our doctors, however, eat alone at their desks or with colleagues, often at informal business meetings. Soups, meat or fish sandwiches, salads, coffee, skim milk, fruit or—more normally—no dessert are almost invariably the menu. Not one doctor we interviewed had a cocktail for lunch.

By evening our experts, not surprisingly, are without exception pretty hungry. Looking in on their dinner hour, you might not spot much at first glance that would strike you as unconventional, but by now we are all aware that there are plenty of differences between the habits of the doctors' families and those of most sedentary middle-class white-collar Americans— enough differences, in fact, to give us critical clues to the secret of staying trim without being swept into the feast-and-famine cycle of dieting that has become so drearily familiar in many households.

Quite possibly you might have spotted the doctor and his wife having *a* cocktail. Most likely it would be Scotch, or bourbon, or gin with low-cal tonic. Most of the men who do have predinner drinks have given up martinis because they are relatively high in calories. At dinner you would most likely see no wine except on the most festive occasions. There would probably be no bread and butter on the table and no sauces. If there were potatoes at all, they certainly would not be French fried because most doctors' families gave them up. ("The last time we had French fries was ten years ago.") In fact, there would be little or no fried food of any kind. If there was any dessert other than fruit, it would probably be ice cream or sherbet, and it would be mostly for the children. The doctor's wife might have a normal portion, the doctor himself probably much less.

What would be most important, however, would also be least apparent, and that's the careful hold-down on fats and on the sizes of portions.

It's time here to take a deep breath and state with every possible emphasis our doctors' Secret No. 4: *They maintain extremely vehement feelings about all fats.* They tend to fear them with a passion. Better than most families, they know that more than 41 percent of the average American's calories come from fats, while the American Heart Association suggests that 25 to 30 per cent would be vastly healthier. The doctors also know that even a little bit of fat contains a *lot* of calories, so every uneaten ounce of fat is another step toward a trim figure. All of which explains why some doctors go to rather silly-seeming trouble to avoid fat. As we've observed, if there is even the slightest visible chunk of the stuff left on a piece of meat at dinner, for instance, many of these doctors don't just cut it off. They make sure to get it all, even if it means cutting off a trace of meat, too. They may also strip the skin from chicken just because it tends to absorb considerable fat.

Fat control for the dinner table begins when the doctors' wives go shopping. Most of them started to reduce or stop their butter-buying as long as ten or fifteen years ago. Often we were told, "I just don't have it around the house." While there is less of the particularly suspect animal fats in margarine, we should be impressed by the number of doctors' wives who in recent years also cut down on margarine (by far their preferred fat for cooking) because they know it contains exactly as many calories as butter. The same diligence dominates all their shopping. Note, for instance, how most of these wives have cut way down on all cheeses except cottage cheese, and how, when they buy cookies for their children, they usually buy plain ones, not those with rich fillings. But mostly they just buy far less of the popular high-fat items than other wives. We were impressed to see that when these women replenish their supplies of potato chips, they may buy a bag or two per month. Their most unconventional fat-reducing measures, however, concern meat. It is also one of the most important because it's so true that, as Harvard's Dr. Jean Mayer told us: "The American public thinks meat is 'low cal.' " Unfortunately, as Dr. Mayer quickly added: "It isn't."

Most people just don't like to believe that meat is rich in fats, especially the best cuts. This leads us straight to the doctors' secret No. 5: Their wives probably *buy meat less often than any Americans except the very poor.* Although their husbands enjoy excellent incomes, these wives rarely buy porterhouse steak or standing rib roast beef. ("I feel sinful when I get a good steak," said Dr. Stare's wife, Helen.) Some of these wives buy steak only about once every three weeks or even less often. More frequently they buy London broil (flank steak) because it contains less fat than the "better" cuts.

Hamburger is not eactly a special treat in most of the doctors' homes where there are youngsters to be fed. But the doctors' wives know that ordinary hamburger as sold in most stores is very fatty indeed. It is of considerable significance that, almost without exception, these women buy ground round or chuck. Instead of roast beef, they buy sirloin tips or rolled roasts. They know that pork contains a lot of fat, especially in variety meats like hot dogs, and so the doctors' wives don't buy much pork, except perhaps ham. And they try to serve fowl or fish or casseroles based on spaghetti and vegetables as often as family tastes allow.

What surprised us most of all was the quantities the doctors' wives buy. Remember how, at Dr. Hellerstein's Cleveland home, one and a half pounds of hamburger is enough for the doctor, his wife, Mary, and their six children, aged three and a half to fourteen? How a two-pound meat loaf lasts not only for dinner but usually yields sandwiches the next day? How Mrs. Ivan Frantz in Minneapolis buys a five-pound rolled roast and makes it last for two meals, even though there are five sons in the family, aged eight through twenty-one?

The same principle applies particularly to such optional items as snack foods. These tempters do not become *excessive* temptations in the homes of our doctors simply because they are not kept in the house all the time, and when they are, they aren't available in seemingly unlimited quantities.

No doubt you noticed that the doctors and their families tend to practice partial self-denial by taking a nibble where most of us take a mouthful. We also think it's important that, as several told us, they consciously cultivate the habit of eating slowly so they can enjoy it more. ("The majority of people I know who are seriously obese are fast eaters.") Even more important, the doctors feel that to waste a certain amount of rich food is nowhere near as sinful as loading it into an overfed body. Many of them, consequently, have worked hard to develop enough willpower to *taste* rich foods, but not to feast on them. ("That dreadful, ridiculous habit of 'cleaning up your plate!' ")

To many a doctor, the act of passing up food when it is already inviting him from his plate is a routine experience, and he doesn't do it only at official functions (where he is quite likely to eat half or less of the servings). He does it at home, too. Typically, when we asked Dr. Henry Janowitz, head of the Division of Gastroenterology at New York's Mount Sinai Hospital, about his dinner that evening, he mentioned, along with such other fare as honeydew melon, "I had one third of a sweet potato."

The concept of nibbling is especially applicable to desserts. Indeed, the doctors' attitude towards desserts must definitely be labeled Secret No. 6. Very few doctors demonstrate the discipline and disdain of Harvard's Dr. Mayer, who not only said, "I avoid them like the plague," but who has also been able to transmit his anti-dessert prejudices to his five children. We think it's worth remembering how, when we peeked into the Mayer refrigerator, we found the scraggly remains of a quart box of cherry vanilla ice cream and heard Dr. Mayer's wife Elizabeth explain, "That was there when we left for the seashore a month ago." Again, it's moderation that matters. ("There's nothing wrong with ice cream. It's a matter of how often you use it"—Dr. Hellerstein.)

Our doctors' families also bake—and even eat!—cake and pie. Again, however, these are only occasional delicacies, though somewhat more frequently served in families where liquor (the other principal source of *optional* calories) is considered unimportant as a source of comfort. You must have observed how rigorously portion control is practiced in the cake-and-pie department in these homes. Surely it's no accident that, in the home of Dr. Reuben Berman, president of the Minnesota Heart Association, the doctor cuts the pie himself, and always makes sure that it yields eight to nine wedges. Dr. Joseph A. Johnston, pediatrician-in-chief at Detroit's Henry Ford Hospital, reported, "We had cake at home last night, but I had it cut so thin it almost fell apart." On the other hand, Dr. Johnston, tense and on the run all day, relaxes with two martinis before dinner and two rye highballs before bedtime.

"It's a damned sight better than Seconal," he said, and quite a few other doctors in our survey enjoy their liquor late at night and for the same reason.

Surprisingly, when we visited the doctors at home around the dinner hour, we almost never felt that austerity was king. Almost all the wives enjoy cooking. Somehow it's encouraging that, even though Mrs. Philip White's husband is the American Medical Association's slimness expert, she is renowned in her social set for her lasagne and chicken chop suey. We enjoy thinking of Dr. Helen Brown, director of dietary research at the Cleveland Clinic, puttering with her chicken tarragon and her sautéed rice. And we should record for the record that Mrs. Henry Taylor, whose husband is professor of physiology at the University of Minnesota and second-in-command to Dr. Ancel Keys, gave us a loaf of just about the best homemade bread we ever ate.

The atmosphere at the doctors' dinner table tends to be talkative and relaxed. A few doctors use the décor more or less to camouflage the fact that there might be more food on the table. ("My wife spends time on table setting, the linen, the color of the flowers and such things.")

And we were intrigued to discover that most of these families talk about almost anything at dinner except food. Again and again the doctors told us, "We never say, 'My, doesn't that look good'" or "We've got so many other things to talk about."

Could it really be that the less you dwell verbally on food, the less you'll eat of it? We think it's entirely possible. It certainly seemed to work that way in many of these families. The exceptions only demonstrated once again that individual variations within the Doctors' Diet can be as drastic as the differences between the doctors' personalities—as long as the doctors' Secret No. 7 is not violated: *the total amount of consumed food and liquor must not cause a weight gain.* As long as you keep this rule in mind, you can live like that famous gourmet Dr. Ancel Keys, who wrote that gourmet cookbook with his wife Margaret and served us one of the candlelight dinners that have acquired for him such a tasty reputation among the doctor's colleagues. ("When I'm faced with dinner without wine, it's like some sort of punishment.")

In almost all the homes of the doctors we visited, we discovered that the fathers, mothers and children eat three somewhat different diets. Yet the variations almost never require separate shopping or separate cooking for any member of the family. More or less unconsciously, these families live by three medically accepted principles: (1) Intensely busy males in sedentary jobs run a relatively high risk of heart disease if they are overweight, especially when they are middle-aged or older, so for them trimness is a vital health measure. (2) Housewives work about as hard as most factory workers and keep longer hours and their arteries tend to stay in better shape than those of men, at least until after the menopause. (3) It rarely pays to make an issue of food with any child; the best way for him to learn healthy eating habits is by parental example and by simply not keeping foods in the home that the parents don't want him to have. (Very few children go out of their way to cheat on food on a significant scale.)

In general, we found that the males in our sample families ate by far the most restrictive diets. They were also the trimmest. Quite a few of the wives were five or ten pounds over their ideal weights, but even though they indulged themselves more than their husbands, we met not one woman who deserves to be called "fat." Many of the ladies have an egg for breakfast (usually soft-boiled and almost never fried). For lunch they are more likely to fix a salad than to clean up high-calorie leftovers, if there are any. At dinner they are more likely than their husbands to help themselves to seconds. Their biggest problem, naturally, is to keep from excessive nibbling throughout the day. Their principal weapon is keeping busy. The working wives we interviewed were invariably grateful that they more or less naturally escaped the dangers of what one doctor called "not really hunger pangs but boredom pangs." As one of the working women said: "If I were home and smelled dinner cooking, it might be different."

One of the most pleasant surprises we encountered was the relative lack of friction between these parents and their children over food. There were a number of overweight children in our sample, but none was seriously obese, and in almost each case the doctor-father felt that the overweight was a temporary problem of adolescence that the children would outgrow.

A few parents are even beginning to feel a little sorry for their youngsters' Spartan lives. ("I think the kids ought to know what a pumpkin pie is.")

Here, then, is the doctors' eighth secret: *Almost none of these parents take their "enforcer" roles too seriously*. And on those occasions when they did crack the whip, they discovered, like other parents, that it doesn't do much good. So then they usually relaxed like everybody else. While several described their children's eating habits frankly as "bizarre," almost all of these parents do little but attempt to keep the consumption of soft drinks, candy, chocolate and desserts to reasonable levels.

Fortunately, the Doctors' Diet has a way of manifesting itself to children subtly, yet unmistakably. Our best illustration of this principle, perhaps, was Skipper, Dr. Page's fifteen-year-old cat, and how her famous owner switched her to skim milk and other low-fat foods when she was two months old. The doctor's sons never forgot how they asked their father about this change and how he told them that the cat's life was being lengthened by the change.

"We don't propagandize the children," said Dr. George Christakis, assistant dean of the Mount Sinai Medical School, who had sons aged seven, eight, and thirteen. The point is that he doesn't really have to. When we visited Dr. Christakis he was the director of the Bureau of Nutrition of New York City's Department of Health, and the principal purveyor of the famous "Prudent Diet," the most widely accepted regimen designed to prevent heart attacks, mostly by cutting down the total fat intake and substituting polyunsaturated (vegetable) fats for saturated (animal) fats. In the last few years Dr. Christakis halved his egg consumption, doubled his intake of fish and veal and cut down quite a bit on beef. In his home, no child could fail to conclude that Mummy and Daddy don't think highly of animal fats or overeating. Other doctors, who do suspect that the children require indoctrination, keep the lectures low-key.

Dr. Fred Schilling, the medical director of the Continental Insurance Company, whose eight children range in age from six to fourteen, probably went further than any of our experts when he warned his youngsters that fat would make "their pipes rusty." We can well believe it when he reported that ice cream and whole milk had actually become "repulsive" to them!

When doctors decide to get tough with themselves, too, as is occasionally necessary, their methods can be rather forbidding, as we found out in the case of Dr. James M. Hundley, the former Assistant United States Surgeon General who now is executive director of the Institute of Medical Sciences at San Francisco's Presbyterian Medical Center. Not every doctor would approve how Dr. Hundley, when he had gained seventeen pounds within six months and found himself weighing 177 after he stopped smoking, simply decided to cut out lunch and go for a walk instead. Unfortunately for him, he was also one of the few doctors who had not had anything but coffee for breakfast in 25 years.

While the resolute Dr. Hundley learned to live on little more than a normal-sized dinner plus two drinks of bourbon and water to "keep me from nibbling before I go to bed," it seemed to us a pretty draconic way to get back to his normal weight of 160 pounds.

Many doctors frown on meal-skipping, but they are

beginning to show increasing interest in the fairly new idea of dividing the day's meals into six or eight or more small snacks, pioneered by Dr. Clarence Cohn, director of the Division of Nutritional Science at Chicago's Michael Reese Hospital. They are impressed with Dr. Cohn's discovery (and so are we!) that the blood cholesterol levels dropped in most of his experimental snackers, that the psychologists who administered tests to the doctor's guinea pigs found that the snackers were "happier" after they had lived on snacks, and that several snackers reported that while their weight stayed unchanged, their fat had evidently been redistributed by their new eating pattern because their waistlines had shrunk by one to one and a half inches.

As we have seen, the evening hours are a time of temptation even for the most weight-conscious physicians. Of the sixty-six respondents to our questionnaire, thirty-eight said they don't have bedtime snacks, but most of the doctors we met personally do drink or nibble after dinner. Dr. Keys's idea to keep two little plastic boxes on his bedside table (one with almonds, the other with dried apricots) struck us as a good one. And we found it refreshing when the University of Minnesota's Dr. Frantz confessed that peanuts and cookies are his weakness. "I'm liable to eat all through the evening. That's my worst sin." The crucial factor in the doctors' night-eating adds up to their Secret No. 9: *they don't fool themselves about it;* they know "it counts," and a night-eater must leave room during the day for any evening "sinning."

The same principle of pay-as-you-go applies to all culinary excesses. Most of our doctors relax about their eating and drinking on weekends, and almost all admit to major caloric splurges on festive occasions (fifty-five of our questionnaire respondents did). But they have learned not to indulge in excesses often enough for the calories to mount up during a typical week. Almost always, they accomplish this "averaging-out" just from habit, although some have developed special ways to "pay" for particular indulgences. You may have been surprised that several of our doctors are fond of beer, but no doubt you also noted that they almost never have it unless they've been doing heavy yard work. And let's not forget that when Harvard's Dr. Mayer craves a healthy portion of wonderful cheese, therefore, he makes a *whole meal* of jellied consommé, cheese, bread and fruit.

This careful juggling of optional foods and drinks also allows the doctors at least occasionally to enjoy "forbidden" items that, in the Doctors' Diet, have been elevated to the rank of delicacies: fried potatoes, potato salad, bacon, doughnuts and, of course, desserts. And for particularly insistent hunger pangs (fifty-four of our questionnaire respondents admitted they have them), they use such appetite depressants as soup, fruit, water, up to 20 cups of coffee a day, and, rarely and invariably to their great regret, tobacco.

It did not take us long to identify another key to the Doctors' Diet: Their ability to practice moderation in the face of the same problems experienced by us members of the Overweight Society is largely a matter of willpower. Willpower, as most of us steady dieters know from long experience, is the key to the doctors' tenth secret: *motivation*. And motivation can be reinforced by information.

It is no coincidence that almost all doctors have truly accepted the regrettable fact that overweight, especially if combined with elevated blood pressure and blood cholesterol levels, shortens life. And it is also no coincidence that the doctor in our sample who ate the most restricted diet of all, Dr. Bruce Taylor, the chairman of the Department of Pathology at Evanston Hospital, learned about dieting from human autopsies. He simply became increasingly impressed —and depressed—by the presence of fat deposits within the arterial walls of heart-disease victims, and perhaps this should make an impression on the rest of us as well.

Dr. Taylor's diet (only about ten percent of his calories derive from fats) is definitely not recommended as a general diet. In fact, we even found a few doctors who developed unpleasant stomach symptoms when they tried to cut down to twenty-five percent. But, since recent medical findings firmly link exercise with the health of human arteries, especially in males, most of our doctors do labor hard to translate their eleventh and last secret: They know that *they must try to overcome their distaste for artificially created physical exertion.*

It's well worth our while to recall how Dr. Taylor walks his beagle two miles a day and mails his letters one at a time so he has an excuse to make more trips to the mailbox; how Dr. Mayer walks an hour to get to his club for lunch and back to his office; how Dr. Stare plays tennis regularly and often finds a sensible reason to take a very fast walk; how Dr. Alexander does exercises in bed for fifteen minutes in the morning and not only walks to his office (a mile each way), unless it rains, but clutches his briefcase for a final 400-yard fast run through the park on the way home; how Dr. Stamler does five minutes of daily calisthenics, never takes the elevator to his fourth-floor office and swims at the "Y" several evenings a week; how Dr. Page plays tennis and exercises in the shower daily before dinner; and how Dr. Hundley does calisthenics after dinner in the basement with his seventh-grade son.

Many of our doctors rarely take elevators for less than four or five flights of stairs, and several told us they try, whenever practical, not to pick up the phone but walk a little to see in person whomever they wanted to contact. Clearly nobody would bother to accept—much less to invite—such inconveniences without very powerful motivation indeed. And in this department, we must admit, the doctors enjoy a few special advantages. To begin with, at many of the professional functions where these men officiate, it just would never do to show up without a trim waistline. After all, a fellow can hardly cut a fine figure as a diet expert and appear overweight before his patients, students, friends and fellow experts. Furthermore, our man is not likely to be a busy doctor and at the same time a phlegmatic, physically inactive person. And it obviously helps that he is better informed than most of us; one reason why he needn't actually count calories is that he knows enough about the caloric values of, say, cake frosting to realize that a few spoonfuls of dessert, when taken daily, can mount up just enough to sweep him into the insidious cycle of creeping weight gain.

Yet what of it? The professional motivations of our doctors—or so we became convinced—are a relatively unimportant factor in their dietary lives. Self-interest, the desire to feel well and live a long life free from disease, is unquestionably what motivates them by far the most strongly. The chances are that you yourself share this attitude with our doctors, for otherwise you would almost certainly not be reading this book.

25

Living with the Doctors' Diet

There is no point in pretending that all the doctors whose habits we surveyed live cheerfully and obediently in accordance with the ground rules that are being followed, by and large, among the professionals who figure in the case histories that we have just examined. As we noted earlier, quite a few of the sixty-six members of the American Society for Clinical Nutrition who responded to our questionnaire had chosen to do little or nothing even about their consumption of such items as eggs, butter and bacon.

Here now are some further results of this survey, some of them surprising:

Fifty-nine of these sixty-six experts now weigh less than their all-time top weight, but twenty-one had never checked their blood cholesterol level and only twenty-six were able to report their 1960 and their 1965 readings (only three reported higher readings);

Forty had changed over to leaner cuts of meat in recent years, but only seventeen reported that they had decreased their beef consumption and forty-three had not increased the amount of fish they eat (which was a real surprise to us!);

Thirty increased their use of skim milk, but twenty-nine reported that they did not;

Thirty decreased their pork consumption, but thirty-four said they did not;

Thirty-five decreased their consumption of commercially baked goods, but twenty-six specified that they did not;

Thirty-five cut down on snack foods, but twenty-five reported that they did not;

Twenty-eight increased their physical exercise, but twenty-nine did not;

Twenty-seven reported that they ate less cheese, but thirty-five reported no change;

Twenty-one changed their salad dressings (mostly to oil and vinegar or low-calorie dressing), but eighteen did not, and an unusually large number of doctors (twenty-three) failed to answer the question because they evidently did not consider it important enough to bother with;

Twenty-nine no longer use sugar, but 34 said they did (only 15 reported that they used artificial sweeteners);

Thirty-six have become more careful in recent years about trimming all visible fats off meat, but twenty-five did not (five said they had always been careful);

Twenty-three reported no change in their consumption of alcoholic beverages, but twenty-two increased their intake, and only two decreased it (seventeen said they don't drink, and two did not report on this point);

As to their wives, only twenty-six of the doctors reported that their ladies ate the same diet as the men (twenty-one said their wives ate a *less* restricted diet, and sixteen reported their wives were eating a *more* restricted diet).

As far as we know, ours is the most intensive inquiry that has yet been launched into the diet changes of qualified nutrition experts, but we would be the last to claim that it constitutes conclusive scientific evidence. Some of the thirty-five doctors who reported no change in their cheese-eating, for example, may well have been eating very little cheese all along. It is also conceivable that some of the twenty-nine doctors who said that they had not increased their exercise in recent years have been doing an hour of calisthenics a day since early childhood. In general, however, we believe that we obtained a reasonably accurate over-all picture of a group of men struggling earnestly with a problem that they consider truly important to themselves.

There were some, of course, who were not doing as well as they might. Dr. C. Frank Consolazio of Fitzsimons General Hospital in Denver, for instance, was clearly overweight at the time of our survey, when he was 52. He weighed 200 pounds (his height is five feet eight and a half inches). He had weighed exactly the same five years before and had at one time weighed as much as 225. He estimated that he ate three thousand calories a day, 40 percent of them derived from fats (the same as five years before). He did not report on his blood cholesterol. He told us that he had cut down "materially" on cheese, "drastically" on whole milk, "slightly" on bacon and that he ate only one egg a week. However, he had not cut down on butter or snack foods, and he enjoyed a daily bedtime snack of "ice cream and a soft drink." His comment will ring true to every one of us dieters:

"My family and I love to eat. This is one expenditure where we do not restrict ourselves. I frequently

go on a weight-reducing diet. During this time I usually omit the noon meal completely and attempt to
increase my physical activity."

There were some lucky fellows who had made very
few changes but who evidently did not need to do
anything at all drastic. One of these is Dr. Edgar S.
Gordon of the University of Wisconsin School of Medicine, who is perhaps the best-known advocate of systematic snacking for obese patients. Dr. Gordon is not
a six-snacks-a-day man himself. All he has for lunch
is an apple and a glass of skim milk, and at bedtime
he has a "snack" consisting of another glass of skim
milk. But the rest of his meals are remarkably conventional. Some 45 percent of his calories come from
fats, according to his own surprising estimate. He eats
six to eight eggs a week and has not cut down on ice
cream, Roquefort cheese salad dressing, bacon, pork
and snack foods.

On the other hand, he eats a total of only 2,000
calories a day (just one hundred in alcohol, and he
almost never eats desserts) and his exercise includes
not only regular sessions of tennis but also three to five
miles of walking *every day*. As a result, this fifty-
seven-year-old physician (his height is five feet seven
and a half inches) weighs only 148 pounds, compared
with 152 pounds five years previously and an all-time
top weight of 164. And his blood cholesterol level is

an exemplary 192 (compared with an equally excellent 205 five years before).

We also heard from doctors who were afflicted with long-standing diet problems and who had tackled them successfully but at a rather late stage and not without considerable difficulty. One of these turned out to be a particularly prestigious pioneer researcher on cholesterol, Dr. Lawrence W. Kinsell of Highland-Alameda County Hospital in Oakland, California.

This scientist (age fifty-nine; height six feet one) had weighed as much as 198 pounds at one time. In the past five years he had been able to control it at a steady (and highly respectable) 185 pounds. However, five years ago his blood cholesterol level was very high indeed: in excess of 350. It is now in the normal range, fluctuating between 190 and 240. However, he admits to suffering hunger pangs "often." His average daily intake in alcoholic drinks is three hundred calories, and his yen for such favorites as lobster, steak and wine continues unabated. Dr. Kinsell has cut down "drastically" on butter, margarine, whole milk, skim milk, pork, baked goods and eggs (he now eats two a week). He also cut down "materially" on beef, cheese and bacon. Eating at restaurants remains a problem for the doctor.

How does he cope with it?

"I do the best I can," he reported.

Another diet expert who healed himself was Dr. O.

Neal Miller of Tulane University. At the age of forty-six (he is six feet tall), Dr. Miller reported his weight at a very trim 171 pounds and his blood cholesterol level at 185. Five years previously his cholesterol had been 265 and his weight 195. Some years earlier he had weighed as much as 210 pounds.

Dr. Miller said he suffered hunger pangs "often," but that he had succeeded in knocking the fat content of his diet from its previous level of 40 percent down to about 20 percent. He had cut down "drastically" on such items as snack foods, bacon and whole milk. He had "materially" reduced his consumption of baked goods and eggs (down to two per week, always boiled). He stopped eating ice cream and chose to eat any kind of dessert only "on occasion."

Here is what this once overweight doctor told us about the way he has by now been able to *keep* down his weight for years: "My success in controlling my weight has been due to my persistent attention to it. I weigh every morning as soon as I get up, dressed the same way. This focuses my attention to the problem. After one has gained five pounds is a little late. The notches on one's belt are not sensitive enough. If I have gained more than a pound, I watch my consumption that day."

Are there still a great many diet experts and other doctors today who eat too much and exercise too little?

Of course there are. In fact, it is time to confess that we were rather shocked to find so many experts who do not practice what they preach. Perhaps we shouldn't have been, because the long-documented truth is that doctors in general take notoriously poor care of themselves. Under the title, "Physician, Heal Thyself," for example, the *Journal of the American Medical Association* in 1962 reported on a survey comparing the true health status of five hundred supposedly "well" business executives with the condition of sixty-eight "well" physicians and dentists. The doctors did not do themselves proud!

"The total number of diseases requiring treatment in the physicians' group averaged 38 percent as compared with 23.9 percent in the executives," the survey found. Moreover, "many more physicians than executives needed treatment not only for new conditions but also for those known to be present beforehand."

Another illustration: Of the 1,759 physicians who submitted to health checks that were offered to them at the 1965 annual convention of the American Medical Association, 1,249 turned up with one or more abnormalities. Leading the list of the most common abnormal conditions that were found in these doctors (in 762 cases!) were blood cholesterol levels of 250 or over.

When it comes to the business of taking *preventive* steps for better health, such as taking off weight or cutting down on dietary fats, the general performance of doctors as a group is even more dismal.

"I see a great many doctors," said Dr. Fred J. Schilling, the medical director of the Continental Insurance Company, "and few have taken off weight. There's been some impact, but I don't think it's of real significance."

Dr. Seymour Rinzler, the cardiologist in charge of the Prudent Diet program in the New York City Department of Health, was even more vexed. He told us of attending a conference on vascular problems. There were about 30 physicians present. Dr. Rinzler asked them how many were following the precepts of the Prudent Diet. Three raised their hands. Then he asked the doctors how many of them would prescribe the Prudent Diet to a patient who has had a heart attack. They all raised their hands.

"How silly!" Dr. Rinzler told us. "After a first heart attack half the patients are gone. The Prudent Diet is a preventive step, but doctors don't seem to understand prevention."

The real point is that doctors are human. Unless they are as fully informed and as deeply convinced as many of the specialists whom we have met in these pages, doctors are like the rest of us and tend to follow the line of the least resistance. Unless patients are grossly obese or otherwise acutely in need of diet-and-exercise therapy, many doctors do not like to burden their own overworked lives by trying to persuade these people to swim against strong cultural tides—and against their own appetites. Fashions and health fears notwithstanding, we are quite literally still living in a fat society. Isn't it true that restaurants still find it good business to promote dishes prepared with "country-fresh butter"? Isn't it still a fact that words like "rich," "thick" and "creamy" are adjectives that attract typical American eaters, rather than repel them? And that the very notion of "eating lean" is only beginning to be understood?

The doctors we have met in these pages, then, are pioneers. They deserve to be admired and imitated. As we have attempted to show, the latitude in *styles* of eating is rather generous as long as total calorie consumption is kept *down* and exercise is kept *up*. The doctors have shown us a surprising variety of simple ways to integrate the prudent life into the daily routine. Perhaps it is naïve at this stage to point out again that you can hardly be tempted during the all-important evening hours by food that is not kept around the house in the first place (we have found that few people really enjoy having to "sneak" food). The practical truth of the matter is that such a reminder is not naïve at all, and a look into your own refrigerator may convince you. Nor is it a waste of time to point out again that it is pretty much impossible for most people to eat their cake and have their liquor, too. Most of us simply do not devote enough attention to the "choice-making" that is required when it comes to the optional "fun" calories in desserts and/or cocktails. Yet the necessity to make such choices is a fact of life. So is the wisdom of certain substitutions, and we would like to sum up some of the simple switches that impressed us as useful and sensible when we visited the homes of some of our diet experts.

Most of them did eat potatoes, but they had them baked, not fried.

They did eat eggs, but rarely, and they ate them poached, not fried or scrambled.

They did nibble on snack foods, but more likely on ginger snaps or oatmeal cookies, not potato chips.

They did like to "fill up" sometimes, but they filled up with coffee, clear soup or water, not fattening items.

They did eat sherbet, but not much ice cream.

They did eat other desserts, but not all the time, and they chose fruit over cake.

They did use milk in their coffee, but not cream.

They did eat cheese, but not so much, and they tried to stick to cottage cheese and other lean varieties.

They did drink liquor, but more likely a highball, not a martini.

They did eat steak, but not the best and fattiest cuts.

They did enjoy food, but eating was not a key interest in their lives.

Finally, let's take another look at the dozen strategic secrets of the Doctors' Diet—the critical steps taken by the best-informed, most up-to-date nutrition specialists and their families. The adults in these families

1. keep watching their weight *all* the time
2. eat relatively small breakfasts and lunches
3. keep busy and unbored
4. cut down on all fats
5. eat less meat than most people and buy smaller quantities of food
6. nibble, especially when it comes to desserts
7. watch their *total* food and drink intake
8. don't badger their children about eating habits
9. don't fool themselves that some of their "sinning" doesn't "count"—it does
10. know that the risks of overeating and under-exercising are real, and their motivation is therefore strong
11. try to overcome their distaste for manmade exercise.

None of this is easy. But it works.

INDEX

Adolescence, 20, 65, 66, 232

Alcoholic beverages, 25–26, 33, 36, 44, 53, 54, 63, 71, 81, 89, 96, 101, 108, 117, 123, 141, 143, 148–149, 159, 160, 166, 168, 171, 176, 181, 187, 197, 205, 210, 212, 222, 223, 228, 229, 234, 242, 244, 245, 250

Alexander, Dr. Benjamin, 42–48, 221, 238

Alexander, Judy, 47–48

Alexander, Marie, 42–45, 47, 48

Alexander, Robert, 48

A.M.A. (See American Medical Association)

American Heart Association, 93, 132, 210, 217, 223–224

American Medical Association (A.M.A.), 58, 59, 64, 216, 229, 247–248

American Society for Clinical Nutrition, 14, 240

American Society of Arteriosclerosis, 129

"Anti-Coronary Club," 173ff., 185, 187, 188, 195

Appetite, 34, 44, 50, 51, 75, 86, 122, 222, 249

Appetite-depressants, 60, 63, 170, 217, 221, 236, 250

Arteriosclerosis, 185–186

Bacon, 27, 35, 51, 62, 81, 88, 117, 147, 169, 188, 195, 204, 220, 226, 236, 240, 244, 245, 246

Baked goods (See Bread, Cake, Cookies, Crackers, Rolls, Toast)

Beans, 69, 71, 79

Beef, 24, 40, 54, 80, 89, 96, 107, 123, 150, 154–155, 168, 175–176, 188, 204, 208, 225, 233, 241, 245

Beer, 26, 50, 63, 124, 178, 197, 236

Berman, Isabel, 141, 142–143

Berman, Dr. Reuben, 139–143, 228

Beth Israel Hospital (New York City), 43, 174

Between-meals snacks (See Snacks)

Blood pressure, 15, 117, 129, 136, 237

Boston *Globe,* 33

Bread, 23, 25, 33, 45, 48, 50, 52, 53, 65, 69, 70, 81, 82, 88, 90, 91, 94, 95, 97, 101, 110, 118, 134, 141, 142, 161, 166, 170, 196, 223, 236, 241, 246 (See also Rolls, Toast)

Breakfast, 22–23, 34, 35, 44, 46, 61, 80, 87, 90, 96, 100–101, 109–110, 116, 119, 123, 124, 133–134, 141, 143, 147, 159, 168, 170, 171, 176, 177, 188, 196, 204, 219, 220–222, 231, 251

Broiling, 53, 169

Brown, Dr. Helen, 121–125, 165, 229

Brown, John, 123ff.

Brown, Peggy, 124

Butter, 22–23, 26, 33, 35, 39, 41, 44, 45, 62, 65, 81, 88, 91, 105, 109, 116, 118, 128, 134, 140, 141, 143, 146, 147, 148, 152, 155, 161, 166, 168, 170, 175, 176, 186, 220, 221, 223, 224, 240, 245 (See also Margarine)

Buttermilk, 81

Cakes and pies, 34, 45, 56, 62–63, 66, 88, 89, 91, 97, 109, 110, 117, 135, 136, 140, 145, 147–148, 149, 155, 156, 171, 176, 180, 187, 189, 199, 228, 241, 246, 250

Calisthenics (See Exercise)

Calories, 11, 22, 24, 25, 32, 36, 50, 51–52, 63, 67, 70, 86, 90, 95, 116, 117, 118, 122, 132, 134, 140, 143, 146, 148–149, 162, 167, 170, 190, 210, 214, 220, 221, 223–224, 236, 239, 244, 249

Canadian Air Force exercises, 63, 171, 207

Canadian bacon, 134

Candy, 40, 41, 82, 88, 91, 134, 143, 154, 163, 171, 172, 199, 232

Carbohydrates, 53, 95, 212

Cereal, 34, 35, 70, 87, 96, 124, 134, 147, 148, 177, 178, 196, 204, 221

Cheese, 23, 24, 37, 44, 46, 51, 70, 71, 80, 81, 89, 90, 94, 98, 101, 110, 128, 133, 147, 152, 156, 159, 160, 168, 176, 186, 187, 195, 208, 224, 250 (See also Cottage cheese)

Chicago Board of Health, Heart Disease Central Section, 214

Chicken (See Poultry)

Chocolate, 45, 82, 136, 163, 166, 183, 199, 232

Cholesterol level, 15, 35, 46, 50, 68–70, 86, 94, 95, 104–105, 123, 128, 129, 146, 154, 161–162, 175, 177, 184, 185, 188, 189, 205, 219, 235, 237, 241, 244–245, 246, 247

Christakis, Emmy, 176, 180ff.

Christakis, Dr. George, 173–183, 194, 233

Christakis, John, 180, 181–182

Christakis, Michael, 180, 181–182

Christakis, Paul, 180, 181–182

Cigarettes (See Smoking)

Cleveland Clinic, 93, 95, 121, 165, 217, 229

Cleveland Heart Society, 129

Clinical Aspects of Arteriosclerosis, The, 186

Coffee, 22, 37, 51–52, 61, 70, 71, 87, 89, 90, 96, 100, 101, 117, 119, 123, 134, 141, 143, 146, 159, 160, 168, 169–170, 177, 187, 188, 196, 217, 220, 221, 222, 234, 250, 251

Cohn, Dr. Clarence, 84–91, 235

Cohn, Pauline, 85ff.

Cola drinks (See Soft drinks)

Consolazio, Dr. C. Frank, 243–244

Consommé, jellied, 24, 236

Continental Insurance Company, 192, 234, 248

Cookies, 44, 66, 81, 94, 95, 101, 110, 112, 118, 124, 142, 156, 170, 181, 198, 224, 235, 250

Corn, 88, 141, 146

Cornell University Medical School, 43

Cottage cheese, 24, 46, 70, 88, 95, 101, 107, 110, 116, 119, 154, 204, 224, 236, 241, 242, 245, 250

Crackers, 37, 71, 81, 96, 119, 123, 124, 148, 159, 160, 198

Cream, 72, 96, 146, 250

Dairy products (See Butter, Cheese, Cottage cheese, Cream, Ice cream, Milk, whole, Skim milk)

Dessert, 21, 34, 40, 45, 54, 62, 66, 71, 80, 81, 89, 91, 97, 117, 122, 134, 136, 141, 145, 149, 152–153, 159, 169, 176, 187, 205, 206, 223, 227–228, 232, 236, 239, 244, 246, 250, 251

Diet foods, 210

Diet pills, 210

Diet-Health Study, 51, 93, 114–115

Diets, 39, 50, 67ff., 70, 173, 174–175, 186, 190, 211 (See also Doctors' Diet, Eating habits, Emotional factors, Motivation, Overeating, Portions, Prudent Diet)

Digestion, 132, 238

Dinner, 33, 45, 53, 65, 71, 80, 88, 91, 96, 101, 107–108, 117–118, 123, 134ff., 141, 148, 156, 159, 177–178, 186, 196, 204–205, 219, 222–223, 224, 229–230, 231

Doctors' Diet, 14–15, 211ff., 216, 218ff., 232, 236ff., 240–251

Doctor's Wife's Thinking Thin Cookbook, The, 82

Eat Well and Stay Well, 106

Eating habits, 59, 60, 69ff., 75ff., 84, 87, 94, 100, 103, 107ff., 116ff., 121ff., 128ff., 133ff., 140ff., 144ff., 150ff., 158ff., 163, 165ff., 175ff., 180ff., 185ff., 188ff., 193ff., 197ff., 209, 215, 218ff., 227, 231, 232, 235ff., 241–242, 249, 249–251

Eggs, 23, 34, 35, 44, 45–46, 51, 52, 61, 69, 70, 77, 87, 94, 98, 101, 109–110, 116, 123, 128, 129, 134–135, 142, 147, 154 155, 159, 168, 170, 176, 180, 188, 195, 198–199, 204, 208, 212, 215, 219–220, 221, 231, 233, 240, 244, 245, 246, 250

Emotional factors, 40, 75ff., 86, 90, 132, 178–179, 235

Evanston Hospital, 67, 237

Exercise, 17, 19, 20–21, 27, 37–39, 44, 46–47, 50, 55, 55–56, 63, 66, 72, 82, 99, 100, 112–113, 118–119, 124, 126ff., 129–130, 131ff., 137, 142, 143, 145, 149, 153, 160–161, 162–163, 166–167, 171, 179–180, 189, 197, 206–207, 211, 214, 216, 238–239, 241, 242, 249, 251 (See also Sports, Walking)

Fat, body, 86, 128, 235, 237 (See also Obesity, Overweight)

Fat deposits (See Cholesterol level)

Fats, animal, 19, 22ff., 35, 45, 46, 50, 52, 57, 62, 67–70, 71, 72, 88, 94, 104–105, 109, 115, 117, 123, 132, 140, 143, 146, 150, 153, 154, 173, 174, 176–177, 182, 186–187, 188, 194, 204, 220, 223ff., 233, 237, 242, 244, 246, 248, 250, 251

Fats, dairy, 39, 46, 51

Fats, vegetable, 173

Fish, 23–24, 33, 35, 45, 52, 53, 56, 62, 70, 77, 80, 96, 110, 116, 117, 129, 141, 148, 154, 168, 175, 177, 178, 188, 195, 196, 204, 206, 222, 226, 233, 241 (See also Seafood)

Fitzimons General Hospital (Denver, Colo.), 243

Food and Agriculture Organization, 20

Food and Drug Administration, 145, 214

Food (See specific foods)

Frantz, Dr. Ivan S., 114–120, 235

Frantz, Veronica, 117ff., 226

"Free eaters," 86

French fried potatoes (See Potatoes)

Fried foods, 39, 43, 45, 53, 88, 198, 223

Fruit, dried, 111, 171, 235

Fruit, fresh, 23, 24, 26, 37, 44, 48, 52, 65, 80, 81, 87, 89, 90, 91, 96, 101, 117, 133, 137, 143, 152, 169, 176, 178, 190, 199, 205, 222, 223, 237, 250

Gelatin, 80, 81, 152

Glenn, Justine, 205ff.

Glenn, Dr. Morton B., 201–208

Gordon, Dr. Edgar S., 244–245

Gravy, 148

Hamburger, 24, 40, 57, 62, 76, 88, 117, 135, 141, 168, 175–176, 190, 196, 225–226
Harris, Flora, 146ff.
Harris, Dr. Philip, 144–149, 214
Harris, Philip Scott, 149
Harvard University, 17–18, 20, 29, 31, 43, 214
Health, 12, 15, 50, 69–70, 77, 86, 135, 151, 153, 194, 213, 231, 238, 247, 249
Heart and artery diseases, 12, 27–28, 31, 50, 68–69, 78, 93, 94, 105, 115, 127, 128, 137, 173–174, 184, 185–186, 220, 231, 237, 248
Heart attack, 69, 77, 174, 185, 219, 233, 248
Hellerstein, Dr. Herman, 126–138, 214–215, 220, 222, 226, 228
Hellerstein, Dr. Mary, 128ff., 226
Henry Ford Hospital (Detroit, Mich.), 228
Highland–Alameda County Hospital (Oakland, Calif.), 245
Hors d'oeuvres, 33, 53, 56
How to Get Thinner Once and for All, 202
Hundley, Dr. James M., 157–163, 234, 238
Hunger pangs, 13, 24, 44, 70–71, 88, 141, 169, 170, 196, 204, 232, 236, 245, 246
Hypertension, 39

Ice cream, 45, 54, 59, 62, 70, 81, 89, 91, 94, 116, 129, 140, 163, 169, 171, 182–183, 195, 223, 228, 234, 244, 250
Ice milk, 116, 205
Indolence, 127, 129
International Society of Cardiology, 105

Jam and jelly, 46, 70, 95, 134, 171, 190, 204, 221

Janowitz, Dr. Henry, 227
Johnston, Dr. Joseph A., 228–229
Jollife, Dr. Norman H., 173–174, 175, 185, 186, 194, 201
Journal of the American Dietetic Association, 165
Journal of the American Medical Association, 247
Juices, fruit, 35, 80, 87, 119, 124, 168, 171, 196, 220 (See also Orange juice)

Keys, Dr. Ancel, 104–113, 114, 214, 229, 230, 235
Keys, Margaret, 106ff., 230
Kinsell, Dr. Lawrence W., 245

Lamb, 99, 176, 204
Life expectancy, 237
Liquids (See Beer, Coffee, Juices, fruit, Milk, whole, Skim milk, Soft drinks, Tea, Water)
Lisa and David, 74
Low-calorie foods, 79, 205
Low-calorie liquids, 25, 171, 190, 217
Lunch, 35, 36, 44, 52, 61, 65, 71, 80, 95, 96, 101, 117, 123, 124, 134, 141, 145, 147–148, 161, 168, 170, 177, 196, 204, 222, 231, 234, 251

Margarine, 22–23, 35, 39, 44, 45, 46, 62, 87, 91, 123, 129, 141, 146, 176, 182, 188, 195, 196, 204, 208, 221, 224, 245 (See also Butter)
Marmalade, 22–23, 87, 123, 221
Mayer, Elizabeth, 26–27, 33, 228
Mayer, Dr. Jean, 17–28, 33, 225, 227–228, 236, 238
Mayonnaise, 52, 213
Meal-skipping, 234
Meat, 23, 24, 35, 39–40, 46, 49–50, 53, 61, 62, 65, 70, 71, 77, 87, 89ff., 96, 99, 101, 107, 110, 117ff., 123, 124, 135, 141, 148, 159, 161, 168,

Meat, cont.
176–177, 178, 181, 186–187, 195, 208, 222, 225, 241, 245, 250, 251 (See also Bacon, Beef, Fats, animal, Hamburger, Lamb, Pork, Poultry, Sausage, Steak, Veal)
Menopause, 231
Metabolism, 122, 124
Metrecal, 71, 100–101
Michael Reese Hospital (Chicago, Ill.), 84, 90, 235
Milk, whole, 22, 34, 44, 46, 48, 51, 61, 70, 91, 94, 110, 116, 119, 133, 141, 147, 148, 155, 159, 171, 177, 178, 195, 196, 220, 221, 234, 245, 246, 250 (See also Buttermilk, Skim milk)
Miller, Dr. O. Neal, 245–247
Minnesota Heart Association, 139, 228
Minnesota School of Public Health, 105
Minnesota, University of, 229, 235
Moderation, 237
Motivation, 31, 46, 75ff., 237, 238, 239, 251
Mount Sinai Hospital (New York City), 174n., 227, 233
Munves, Dr. Albert W., 167, 170ff.
Munves, Dr. Elizabeth, 164–172, 214

New York City Department of Health, 173, 194, 201, 233, 248
New York State Dietetic Association, 165
New York University, 165
Nibbling, 84, 85ff., 101, 123, 134, 136, 180, 227, 231–232, 234, 252, (See also Snacks)
North Carolina, University of, 69
Northwestern University Medical School, 68
Nuts, 33, 63, 70, 71, 111, 118, 235

Obesity, 74, 109, 201, 203, 227, 232, 244, 248 (See also Overweight)
Oil, corn, 23, 80, 108, 123, 176, 177, 188, 195, 199
Oil, olive, 176
Oil, vegetable, 39, 53, 110, 156, 180, 181, 198
Oleomargarine (See Margarine)
Optional foods and drinks, 235ff., 250
Oral gratification, 86
Orange juice, 35, 116, 123, 188, 221
Overeating, 232ff., 236, 243–244, 251
Overweight, 11, 19, 31, 74, 76, 80, 90, 129, 149, 164–165, 180, 201, 231, 232, 237, 243 (See also Obesity)

Page, Beatrice, 97ff.
Page, Christopher, 99, 101–102
Page, Dr. Irvine H., 92–103, 217, 233, 238
Page, Nicholas, 99, 101–102
Pasta, 53, 65, 88, 89 (See also Spaghetti)
Peanut butter, 94–95, 102, 133–134, 217
Pie (See Cakes and pies)
Pie crust, 147–148
Pills, diet, 210
Polyunsaturated fats, 23, 177, 233 (See also Fats, vegetable)
Pork, 226, 241, 244, 245
Portions, 24, 33–34, 36, 40, 64, 66, 89, 96, 119, 124, 133ff., 143, 168, 177, 217, 223, 228, 251
Potato chips, 26, 44, 169, 181, 198, 225, 250
Potatoes, 45, 53, 62, 70, 88, 89, 117, 133, 141, 147, 154, 161, 169, 176, 198, 223, 236, 250
Poultry, 35, 45, 46, 52, 53, 65, 89, 101, 110, 123, 129, 135, 148, 168, 176, 188, 196, 204, 224, 226

Presbyterian Medical Center (San Francisco, Calif.), 158n., 234
Protein, 87, 90
Prudent Diet, The, 173ff., 180, 185, 188, 190, 194, 195, 233, 248
Psychological factors (See Emotional factors)
Public Health Service, 158
Puddings, 80, 81, 136

Recipes, 82, 106, 122
Research, 15, 19, 22, 59, 61, 68–69, 85ff., 93, 95, 105–106, 127ff., 139, 154–155, 160, 167, 204, 212–213
Rinzler, Lois, 190, 191
Rinzler, Rita 189ff.
Rinzler, Robert, 191
Rinzler, Dr. Seymour, 184–191, 194, 248
Rolls, 45, 65, 94, 97, 134, 204, 208, 212
Rousseau, Jean-Jacques, 19
Rubin, Eleanor, 76, 78, 81–82
Rubin, Dr. Theodore Isaac, 74–83

Saccharin, 25, 44, 52, 221
Salad dressing, 62, 70, 88, 96, 169, 177, 188, 241–242, 244
Salads, 23, 33, 35, 46, 52, 65, 71, 80, 84, 96, 120, 123, 133, 169, 177, 220, 231
Salt, 39, 117, 136, 169
Sandwiches, 36, 44, 52, 61, 65, 89, 117, 123, 143, 168, 177, 186, 188, 196, 217, 222
Saturated fats, 177, 233 (See also Fats, animal)
Sauces, 36, 53, 108, 109, 223
Sausage, 34, 35, 140, 215, 221
Schilling, Betty, 197ff.
Schilling, Dr. Fred J., 192–200, 234, 248
Seafood, 23–24, 39, 53, 80, 88, 177, 245 (See also Fish)

"Seconds," 33–34, 47, 97, 111–112, 124, 136, 231
Self-denial (See Self-discipline)
Self-discipline, 19, 34ff., 51, 59, 98, 142, 162, 226–227, 233ff., 237
Sherbet, 34, 70, 95, 110, 136, 146, 153, 223, 250
Shopping, 224ff., 230, 251
Skim milk, 34, 61, 65, 69, 70, 81, 87, 90, 95, 96, 101, 107, 110, 116, 123, 133, 134, 153, 154, 169, 177, 178, 194, 195, 196, 204, 208, 217, 221, 222, 241, 244, 245 (See also Milk, whole)
"Smith," Dr., 150–156
Smoking, 60, 64–65, 97, 98, 111, 155, 158–159, 190, 206, 210–211, 217, 234, 237
Snacks, 24–25, 37, 44, 53, 54, 63, 65, 71, 81, 84, 85ff., 88, 96, 111, 117ff., 124, 142, 143, 147, 148, 159, 161, 169, 171, 178, 182, 187, 190, 195, 196, 205, 219, 226, 235ff., 241, 244, 246, 250
Soda pop (See Soft drinks)
Soft drinks, 117, 141 182, 199, 232
Soup, 35, 53, 61, 63, 84, 88, 107, 119, 168, 217, 222, 237, 250
Spaghetti, 76, 89, 133, 188, 226
Sports, 27, 38, 47, 64, 82, 99, 101–102, 112–113, 119, 161, 167, 179, 238 (See also Exercise)
Spreads (See Butter, Margarine)
Stamler, Dr. Jeremiah, 49–57, 213–214, 220, 238
Stamler, Paul, 57
Stamler, Rose, 52, 56
Stare, Dr. Frederick, 29–41, 114, 214, 218, 220–221, 238
Stare, Helen, 31, 34, 37ff., 218, 225
Stare, Mary, 32, 34, 39, 41, 43
Statistics, 20, 105, 174
Steak, 39–40, 62, 76, 80, 88, 123, 135, 141, 148, 190, 195, 200, 205, 250

Sucaryl, 101, 221

Sugar, 25, 35, 44, 51, 61, 143, 146, 152, 153, 159, 178, 196, 242

Surgeon General's Committee Report on Smoking, 158

Tastes in eating, 51, 54, 57, 71, 110, 116, 194, 212, 217-218, 227 (See also Eating habits)

Taylor, Dr. Bruce, 67–73, 128, 132, 237–238

Taylor, Dr. Henry, 229

Tea, 23, 80, 81, 110–111, 112, 119, 143, 160

Teflon utensils, 45, 146, 147

Thin Book by a Formerly Fat Psychiatrist, The, 75

Toast, 46, 61, 70, 87, 119, 123, 124, 133, 143, 168, 170, 188, 190, 204, 221 (See also Bread)

Tobacco (See Smoking)

Tomato, 44, 52, 54, 71, 88, 91, 177, 204

Veal, 45, 80, 110, 169

Vegetables, 22, 33, 65, 69, 71, 72, 79, 118, 141, 148, 175, 181, 182, 226 (See also Beans, Potatoes, Salads)

Waistline, 86, 198, 216, 235, 239

Walking, 21, 38–39, 44, 47, 55, 63–64, 66, 72, 82, 87, 99–100, 112, 130–131, 145, 153, 161, 167, 171, 179–180, 189, 197, 234, 238, 239, 244 (See also Exercise)

Water, 237, 250

Water retention, 39

Weighing, 216

Weight management, 32, 42, 45, 54, 61, 86, 97, 122, 133, 145, 162, 164, 167, 188, 196–197, 203, 216, 245, 246–247, 248, 251

Western Reserve University, 127

White, Chuck, 65, 66

White, Hilda, 64–65, 229

White, Nancy, 65

White, Dr. Philip L., 58–66, 216–217

White House Conference on Health, 161

Willpower, 75

Wine, 33, 44, 53, 89, 108, 166, 178, 205, 223, 245

Winship, Thomas, 33

Wisconsin University School of Medicine, 244

Work, 221–222, 231, 232, 236, 251

World Health Organization, 20, 105

Wyden, Barbara, 32ff.

Wyden, Peter, 32ff.

Yogurt, 170, 180